Your Baby's Best Shot

Your Baby's Best Shot

Why Vaccines Are Safe and Save Lives

Stacy Mintzer Herlihy
and
E. Allison Hagood

ROWMAN & LITTLEFIELD
Lanham • Boulder • New York • London

Published by Rowman & Littlefield Publishers, Inc.
A wholly owned subsidiary of The Rowman & Littlefield Publishing Group, Inc.
4501 Forbes Boulevard, Suite 200, Lanham, Maryland 20706
www.rowman.com

Unit A, Whitacre Mews, 26-34 Stannary Street, London SE11 4AB

British Library Cataloguing in Publication Information Available

Library of Congress Cataloging-in-Publication Data

The hardback edition of this book was previously cataloged by the Library of Congress as follows:

Herlihy, Stacy Mintzer, 1970–
  Your baby's best shot : why vaccines are safe and save lives / Stacy Mintzer Herlihy and E. Allison Hagood.
    p. cm.
1. Vaccination—Popular works. 2. Vaccination of children—Popular works.
3. Immunization of children—Popular works. I. Hagood, E. Allison. II. Title.
RA638.H47 2012
614.4'7—dc23   2012010577

ISBN 978-1-4422-1578-8 (cloth : alk. paper)
ISBN 978-1-4422-1579-5 (pbk. : alk. paper)
ISBN 978-1-4422-1580-1 (electronic)

Printed in the United States of America

Contents

Foreword

$\mathcal{W}$e ask a lot of our citizens.

Children are recommended to receive vaccines to prevent fourteen different diseases in the first few years of life and another two in adolescence. This means that they can receive as many as twenty-six inoculations by the time they're six years old and as many as five shots at one time. No matter how sophisticated a parent might be about vaccines and how they work, it's hard to watch children get so many shots. In many ways, vaccines are the perfect storm of fear; parents see their children get a lot of shots containing ingredients they often don't understand to protect against diseases they don't see; in a sense, vaccines are a victim of their own success. So it's not surprising that some parents are choosing to delay, withhold, separate, or space out vaccines.

Unfortunately, the choice not to get vaccines isn't risk free. In the past few years, outbreaks of measles, mumps, bacterial meningitis, and whooping cough have claimed the lives of many children. Although medicine has limits, preventing certain infections by vaccination isn't one of them. As a doctor, it's particularly hard to watch children suffer something that could have been prevented. And as a parent, whose number one job is to put my children in the safest position possible, it's indefensible to expose them to potentially fatal infections or to expose those with whom they come in contact.

Although several books have been published discussing the science behind vaccines—how they're made, how they work, how they're regulated, what's in them, and their relative risks and benefits—none have been written from the parents' point of view. In *Your Baby's Best Shot*, Stacy Herlihy and Allison Hagood offer something that isn't contained in most vaccine books. Written in clear, easy-to-understand prose, the book provides wonderful information in an empathetic manner. It's an excellent guide to what any new parent can easily perceive as a daunting, almost impossible task: understanding vaccines.

Dr. Paul Offit

Acknowledgments

STACY

This book was an act of love, courage, and sheer determination. I would like to thank the following people for making that daunting task easier.

Diane Volpe Sattler for her kindly encouragement and long years of mentoring. **Tish Davidson** for her useful suggestions about parts of this manuscript and assistance in nagivating the publishing world. **Ann Fisher**, my wonderful ninth grade English teacher who first made me think I could be a writer. **Andrea Delman** for generously sharing her vast knowledge about vaccines and everything else parenting. **Dr. Esther Aronson** for allowing me to pick her brain about this subject and showing me how to write about it both passionately and effectively. Our editors **Suzanne Staszak-Silva** and **Melissa McNitt** for their perceptive editing suggestions. **Dr. Paul Offit** for patiently answering my questions about vaccines and bravely standing up to the pro-infectious disease crowd. **Arthur Allen** for magnanimously sharing his knowledge of all areas of writing. **Phyllis Juried**, my first editor, for helping me learn how to meet a deadline. My coauthor **Allison Hagood** for her unflagging enthusiasm, understated wit, demanding high standards, and love of the Oxford comma.

Brendan Thomas Herlihy Jr.—the best man I've ever met—for his clever mind, loving heart, keen intelligence, insightful ideas, and constant help and support throughout this entire process. And for my very favorite kids: **Serena Jane** and **Charlotte Winifred**. Watching the two of you as you grow up has been an astonishing and constantly unfolding delight.

ALLISON

*W*hen you've been researching, reading about, and discussing an issue for years, it's difficult to adequately acknowledge everyone who's been a part of that process. I can't count how many people have helped me on this journey, nor will I be able to thank every one of those people sufficiently.

Paul Offit, Kathleen Seidel, David Gorski, Seth Mnookin, Michael Shermer, David Myers, Steven Novella, and **Robert Park** have all written books and blogs that have been of invaluable assistance as I investigated the various issues. I am indebted to their hard work and clear thinking.

Our editors, **Suzanne Staszak-Silva** and **Melissa McNitt**, have been incredible. They've been encouraging throughout this process and provided some perceptive advice along the way.

My students throughout the years have been a great source of my development as an educator and writer. As they question me, I learn better ways to explain the complicated concepts contained in this book. If the writing here is helpful to parents, it is because my students taught me how to teach them well.

I appreciate my colleagues' willingness to listen to my thoughts and provide feedback. Special recognition goes to **Christine Swenson, Erica Henningsen Smith, Lori Tigner, Don Walker, Daniel Gore, Rosann Poltrone,** and **Kathryn Winograd**.

My friends have been unwavering sources of support and patience through my years of exploring this issue. I appreciate every single one of them who challenged me, argued with me, disagreed with me, and ultimately stood behind me as I wrote this book. Special thanks to **Bryan Lott, Meta Eaton, Alicia Seveland, Tony Kisling, Virginia Geist, Ben Fontes, Lyon Pound,** and **Joshua Duke** for solid grounding.

My family always believed in me, especially my mother, **Susan Orander.**

Most grateful thanks to **Adam Norman**, who never let me get discouraged, picked me up when things weren't working, and made sure I kept my eye on the right goals. I couldn't have done this without you.

And, finally, my coauthor, **Stacy**, who pulled me into this endeavor, and pushed me to write better than I thought I could. Thanks also to **Brendan, Serena,** and **Charlotte** for letting me take Stacy's attention away from them for so long.

· 1 ·

Who We Are and
Why We Wrote This Book

STACY'S STORY

$\mathcal{F}$rom the moment of the first smallpox inoculation, vaccines have been fodder for societal debate. On the one hand are parents concerned about the thought of injecting their children with something that others have told them might potentially cause harm. On the other are medical professionals attempting to explain exactly why vaccines are safe and save lives.

Vaccines are an issue every single parent must confront nearly instantly. Within hours of birth, most American children are given the first of three shots designed to protect a newborn against hepatitis B. As a baby grows up, doctors in the United States and many nations across the world recommend that parents give their child more than three dozen immunizations.

Mixed in with the voices of pediatricians are the other voices so many parents hear talking about vaccines.

Celebrities such as Jenny McCarthy write best-selling books alleging that vaccines harm children. A single Google query can yield pages of websites filled with allegations that common shots are responsible for modern epidemics of diseases including diabetes, asthma, autism, and childhood obesity.

Reasonable parents can listen to both camps and still not know where to turn.

On December 26, 2002, I gave birth to a child and immediately became that person known as a new mother. New mother as in the last time I held an infant in my arms I was four and the baby in question was my little brother. New mother as in I was grateful for more than an hour of sleep at a time. New

1

mother as in I still wasn't quite sure what to do when my daughter cried or exactly how to give the baby a bath without turning the entire bathroom into a morass of baby toys and sodden towels.

My own mother, glowing in the aftermath of the delight of the birth of her first grandchild, had recently left the baby and me to go back to her condo a dozen states away. She'd given me a five-week apprenticeship in the art of baby caring, but I still felt as unprepared as a college freshman the instant she left.

What actually surprisingly scared me the most was the subject I'd spent hours studying while pregnant: vaccines. Vaccines were all over the news at the time. Everywhere you turned it seemed as if children were getting the measles shot and seemingly instantaneously showing signs of autism. At the same time, my next-door neighbor (a pediatrics nurse) had solemnly told me stories of caring for tiny babies on respirators due to pertussis. A nurse in a neighborhood school had given out vaccine exemptions as easily as one might hand out permission for a school trip, and the resulting eruption of pertussis was traced to that nurse's doorstep.

As a history major I am familiar with the effects of vaccine-preventable illnesses throughout history. Queen Elizabeth I was expected to die of small-pox and bore the scars of her struggle for the rest of her life. Her descendant Queen Victoria lost a grown daughter and several grandsons to diphtheria. FDR, my father's favorite president, nearly died after contracting polio and is famous for serving his presidency in a wheelchair.

I knew all of this and yet and yet and yet . . . I stood on the threshold of the pediatrician's office still worried. Fellow parents had cautiously whispered stories about vaccine reactions during my pregnancy. A few had sat at my baby shower recounting episodes of babies who had their shots and then fell seriously ill a short time later, never to recover.

I wanted to protect my daughter against such diseases in the abstract, but faced with a real-life situation I suddenly was sure but still scared.

I finally plopped my daughter in my lap, stuck a breast in her mouth, and let the pediatrician administer her DTaP needle. Four hours later my daughter started to cry. The crying was normal, but this particular cry had a much uglier sound to it. The sound was high pitched, and it was constant. My daughter seemed to struggle for every single breath, and her howling grew louder and louder with time.

In my panic I lost track of how long her crying fit lasted. It may have been twenty minutes, it may have been an hour, but during that time period my natural parental fear overcame my understanding of the necessity of vac-cines. My daughter's weeping reverberated in my brain. As I rocked her back and forth and my husband frantically sought out the pediatrician's number, I was horrified. The voice in my head started to recount all that I had read about vaccines harming babies. For that brief period of time I became convinced I had made the wrong decision on vaccines. Hours and hours spent reading the anti-vaccine literature had finally completely made me believe that all anti-vaccine people were utterly right.

I felt like the world's worst parent.

Eight years later my daughter is fine. She's more than fine. She reads Terry Pratchett novels. She can multiply three-digit numbers, identify Mongolia on a map, and spend hours exercising to *Dance Dance Revolution* with her father. She's happily enjoying being a big sister.

Today vaccines remain as much in the news as ever. In 2010 the number of whooping cough cases soared, in part because of nonvaccination. A mumps epidemic broke out in Brooklyn. A single unvaccinated child triggered a huge eruption of measles cases in San Diego in 2008.

Vaccines are perhaps the greatest health miracle ever known to mankind. Inoculations will protect babies and toddlers from everything from pneumonia to chickenpox. Vaccines such as the hepatitis B and Gardasil vaccines can actually act as anticancer protection by greatly reducing the odds of getting liver or cervical cancer.

As late as even a century ago a woman wasn't considered a "real mother" until she had lost at least one baby to illness. Most parents today barely give measles or rubella a first thought let alone a second or third thought.

Yet as vaccines have become widely available and in much greater use, so too have voices raised against them become louder and louder in the public square.

Parents like me are often left full of questions even if we choose to vaccinate. I hope this book will help to answer such questions. I hope that anyone reading this book will gain an understanding of why vaccines are so vitally important to the health and well-being of all of us.

I'd like to think this is the book I wanted when my daughter was two months old and in the middle of a vaccine reaction—the kind of book I hope any parent can turn to and walk away with their questions answered and their fears about the subject completely gone.

ALLISON'S STORY

Let's get something out of the way at the beginning.

I do not have children.

This piece of information will automatically cause some readers to dismiss my contributions to this book, and perhaps the book itself. Those readers may think to themselves, "Well, how can she possibly know what it's like to worry about negative side effects of vaccines?"

The answer, of course, is that I cannot, not from personal experience. I can only learn from observing friends and family members go through the process of making hard, important, and lifesaving decisions for their children, and from listening to their discussions of the thought processes behind those decisions. I have watched friends struggle with all sorts of parenting decisions, from vaccinations to school systems to whether or not to buy their girls Barbies. I have engaged in many, many conversations about balancing scientific research with personal opinions and philosophies.

I can also point out that parents often do not expect their pediatrician to have children, and they still can and do accept that the pediatrician is an expert in his or her chosen field. Most people do not wait until their doctors have had a broken leg before being comfortable with having a broken leg treated. People with cancer accept medical advice and treatment from oncologists who've never had cancer. It is not necessary for someone to have personal experience with a situation in order for that person to understand the scientific information regarding that situation.

But what I can and do know is that there is an enormous amount of misunderstanding and misinformation out there regarding science in general, and the science of vaccines in particular. My contributions to this book are designed in some small way to address those gaps in knowledge, so that people making decisions about vaccines can do so with a full understanding of the issue. I want people to have empirical information regarding the science of drug development and the research regarding vaccines. I want to increase people's understanding of the validity of arguments surrounding the vaccine issue. I want people to be able to identify when they are being given misinformation designed to confuse or frighten them.

When it comes to important decisions, many people choose to rely on their gut instinct, their "feeling" about the issue. The most widespread craze in pop psychology today can be phrased as "Trust your gut!" We are told that our instincts, intuition, or gut feelings are the most trustworthy way to understand the world. Follow your heart, say the pop psychology experts, and you'll never go wrong!

They couldn't be further from the truth.

Natural human intuition is loaded with errors in the way we process information from the world around us. Left to our own devices, we will make a number of mistakes when we think about our lives. Most of the time, those errors are inconsequential. Relying on our gut instinct about what restaurant at which to eat, or whether to go to the 7:00 p.m. or 9:00 p.m. movie, doesn't leave us open to large negative consequences if we are wrong. But relying on our gut instinct about complex, complicated issues may very well do just that.

I want parents to be able to make what really is one of the easiest decisions regarding their children's health in an atmosphere of support and comfort, armed with enough background to feel they have made the right decision when they decide to vaccinate their children. Therefore, I wrote this book to help parents recognize the importance of using science and research to make the decision to vaccinate.

In the search for information about the safety of vaccines for their children, parents will inexorably believe they are truly avoiding their own biases and seeking out valid and objective sources of information. Unfortunately, those well-meaning parents will be less successful than they are aware. Everyone falls victim to cognitive biases that limit our ability to accurately gather information unless we are very, very careful. I wrote this book in order to help address the most common biases in the vaccine issue.

Cognitive Biases and You: How They Work, Why They Hurt

We have a tendency to seek out information that confirms our preexisting belief system. We want to believe we are right. This inclination, known as confirmation bias, limits our ability to accurately weigh information about complex issues. It leads us to reject information that tells us we might be incorrect. If a parent has already established a suspicion of medical science, that parent will be more likely to pay attention to stories about possible negative reactions to vaccines. Those stories will not be balanced by context such as the kinds of reactions, how often, out of how many injections, and so on.

It is quite easy, and indeed completely natural, for people who are distrustful of vaccines to seek out information supporting their belief that vaccines (and by extension, doctors, pharmaceutical companies, and scientists) are not to be trusted. There is valid evidence of adverse reactions to vaccines, ranging from mild to severe. Such evidence is used by vaccine doubters to bolster their arguments against vaccines. However, those doubters ignore equally valid (and certainly more abundant) evidence of the benefits of vaccines because of confirmation bias.

Strongly related to confirmation bias is the concept of illusory correlation. This is the belief that two things are related when they are not. An example related to the topic of this book is the often-reported (and scientifically debunked) relationship between vaccines and autism. For reasons that will be explained in later chapters, a single badly designed research study claimed to have found a link between the administration of the measles, mumps, and rubella (MMR) vaccine and autistic symptoms in children. This result, irresponsibly spread by a sensationalist media, became entrenched in parents' minds. Parents of children with autism began to insist they knew immediately that their child was damaged by vaccines, often claiming their child became instantly autistic in the doctor's office. These stories influenced other people to begin "noticing" this illusory correlation.

What went (and continues to go) unrecognized are all the instances in which children receiving vaccines are not diagnosed with autism, or the instances in which children not receiving vaccines are diagnosed with autism. This is an example of the illusory correlation ("vaccines cause autism") working in conjunction with the confirmation bias (noticing only confirming instances).

Humans like stories. We like words that can help us create pictures in our minds of how the world is or should be. We distrust numbers and cold, hard scientific data. We want to hear stories (also called anecdotes) rather than statistics (also called research).

The problem is that easily remembered stories are easily remembered for a reason. Vivid information tends to be unusual or abnormal in some way. When asked about violence in American high schools, Columbine is a vivid case that comes to mind. When asked about violence on American college campuses, Virginia Tech will probably be the one that most people recall. However, neither is a typical example of high school or college violence (thankfully). The extreme nature of these examples makes them memorable and easily recalled, but they are not in any way representative of typical American high schools or colleges.

In terms of this book's topic, emotional cases of parents discussing how their child went from completely normal to 100 percent autistic in an instant after receiving a vaccine are dramatic and emotionally involving. These cases, therefore, are much more memorable than dry statistics regarding vaccine safety, autism development (which does not occur instantaneously), and medical research.

Parents often search for information about vaccines by starting with a search for information on negative reactions (which do occur). When parents find such information, it is more influential on their decision-making process than a piece of information about the positive aspects of vaccines. First, the negative reaction information would tend to be in the form of a story about what happened to a child—emotional, sensational, and attention grabbing. In contrast, the information about the positive aspects of vaccines would more than likely be in the form of a *lack* of stories. Vaccines, after all, prevent illnesses, and it's difficult to make a colorful and attention-grabbing story out of children *not* getting sick or dying of measles. Therefore, the negative information is about rare cases (and usually not placed in context). Parents would naturally be much more able to build a picture of their own child experiencing the same results. It's much harder to build an equally emotional picture of your child being healthy.

Scientific Evidence: The Treatment for Cognitive Biases

Since 1999, I have been teaching college students ranging in age from 17 to 70, and in that time I have witnessed an appalling lack of understanding of science and the scientific method. I have heard students say, "I don't believe in science," as if science were nothing but a philosophy or a religion, with no basis in objective observable fact. These statements often imply that the speakers haven't taken advantage of scientific advancements throughout the course of their lifetimes. Students seem to not understand how science addresses matters of the observable and measurable world, and how that focus doesn't require any sort of belief system.

I have had the same conversations with friends and acquaintances. We seem to view science as something to be distrusted, fought against, or rejected, like some sort of repressive regime designed to reduce our freedom of thought.

In fact, science is not a religion. It is not a belief system. It is a way of taking observations and measurements of the world around us and analyzing those results. The method and analysis that scientists use aren't mysterious rituals, and it's easy for you to understand them. Understanding the scientific method and the reasons for its use allows you to easily identify valid information from misinformation and lies.

Science doesn't replace religion or personal philosophy, and it doesn't strive to do so. People can maintain any sort of personal belief system they want and still be a scientist or simply understand the scientific method and what it can tell us.

My contribution to this book, therefore, is meant to provide parents with some small background in understanding what the science states about vaccines. Parents will always experience worry and fear with regard to the decisions they make on behalf of their children—it is my hope that the information in this book will allow parents to recognize how to make rational decisions based on empirical fact, in spite of the natural concerns they may have regarding those decisions.

It is my hope that this book gives people a better understanding of how scientific research works, how that research applies to the field of vaccines, and what that research tells us about vaccines.

The Edward Jenner Story:
A Brief History of the First Vaccine

$\mathcal{M}$ost medical procedures have been developed more recently than you might think. The first commercial antibiotic dates only to the late 1920s.[1] Chemotherapy was not developed until the middle of the last century. From effective anesthesia to C-sections with low mortality rates to dialysis and bypass operations, many modern medical techniques have been created and refined only within the last fifty years. For a long time a doctor could do almost nothing for a patient other than cut off his rotting limb quickly or help decrease her chances of delivering a baby without dying.

This is not true of vaccines. Vaccines, unlike cosmetic surgery or kidney transplants, aren't a modern medical invention. In fact, vaccination is one of the very oldest known forms of medical treatment. The history of inoculation as a means of protecting people from serious illness dates back many centuries.

Today we have vaccinations against twenty-two diseases. Vaccines for many other diseases are likely to be added in the coming decades. Sixteen vaccines are on the standard vaccine schedule in many countries. One vaccine was on the standard vaccine schedule, but it is used today by only a handful of people in very specific circumstances.

Which vaccine? The vaccine used against smallpox.

For a very long time most vaccination efforts focused largely on that specific disease. Smallpox was the heart of initial vaccine development for a variety of reasons. For one thing, this disease was endemic to many countries rather than just a single place. For another, it struck hard and struck often, killing people in large batches. Smallpox also had a mechanism of transmission that was more easily understood than several equally deadly diseases such as tuberculosis. These characteristics made eradicating the disease or diminishing the effects a huge priority for many communities.

To write about the history of vaccination is to write about the history of smallpox, or variola, as the disease is known in Latin. To write about smallpox is also—amazingly enough—to write about how humanity rid itself of this ancient and not-so-ancient horror. The ravages of smallpox are closer than many people might think. Were you or your parents born in the 1960s? Then you were born in a time when smallpox was still a threat. As late as 1967, smallpox was common in thirty-one countries and infected more than fifteen million people.[2] Over two million died of the disease in that year.[3]

The last known case of smallpox was seen in Africa in 1977.[4] In a single decade a disease that had long terrorized people was finally removed from the world after health officials from various nations banded together and got rid of it. The effort was the culmination of nearly two centuries of investigation, determination, and sheer hard work.

Smallpox derives its name from the size of the pox, or welts, that develop on an infected person's skin. Larger welts often indicated syphilis. A rash from smallpox could spread all over an infected individual's body very quickly. People developed poxes from the rash everywhere including on their eyelids, scalp, and the soft tissue of the mouth and vagina. The start of the disease began with an infectious period of a week or two. After the incubation period had passed, the sufferer would start to feel additional symptoms, including high fevers and headaches. Two to four days later, the disease's hallmark rash would begin. For the next week, people infected with smallpox often became entirely covered from head to toe in a rash of fluid-filled bumps that had a raised indentation resembling a bellybutton.[5] After a time, the pustules would start to scab over and fall off. Unless someone had had smallpox before, during this entire time the patient was contagious and capable of easily spreading the deadly illness to other people.[6]

Once the crusted-over pustules fell off, some of them would leave scars. Many people emerged from a bout of smallpox with horrible side effects. Some had hugely disfiguring scars all over their faces. Others faced the loss of eyesight if the pox spread to their eyes, or the use of an arm or leg if the pox spread to the extremities. Smallpox was responsible for one-third of all blindness cases in eighteenth-century Europe.[7] The only good part about surviving the illness was that survivors could only get it once. Once you recovered from smallpox, you would never get it again.

Historians believe that smallpox started infecting human beings over ten thousand years ago, possibly as a result of our contact with domesticated animals.[8] Smallpox infection has been documented across many cultures. Researchers have been able to find evidence of smallpox in Egyptian mummies dating back three thousand years.[9] Records from ancient China and India have clearly documented cases of smallpox dating back over two thousand years.[10]

Roughly 30 percent of all sufferers who contracted the illness died from it. That was from the most common form known as the ordinary form. Several less common forms, such as the malignant variant of smallpox or the hemorrhagic kind, left only a handful of survivors. The sheer number of people dying is nearly unimaginable to most people today. During the eighteenth century, one child out of every seven died of smallpox in Russia.[11] They were part of a larger ongoing epidemic that claimed over four hundred thousand lives in Europe each year.[12] Many of these deaths were children. Essentially, smallpox would come around every few years and then kill off one in four or one in three kids depending on the severity of the epidemic.

The disease did not distinguish between young and old, rich and poor, or healthy and already sick. Smallpox showed up in periodic outbreaks and hit everyone hard. Cures were futile and treatments essentially nonexistent. The most that people could do was just wait it out and watch the infected person. Very few places on the planet were untouched by the disease. Emperors and peasants, princesses and scientists, little children, adults in the prime of their lives, and the elderly and babies all died when smallpox showed up. Several Russian czars survived, as did Greek historian Thucydides, Lakota Indian chief Sitting Bull, George Washington, Abraham Lincoln, and Andrew Jackson. Five monarchs died from smallpox. Benjamin Franklin lost the youngest of his sons and spent the rest of his life vigorously advocating in favor of the vaccine.[13] Even as recently as 1921, more than one hundred thousand cases of smallpox were recorded in major American cities.[14]

The Americas and Australia remained untouched by the epidemic until the Columbian era. Explorers and colonists are believed to have brought smallpox to natives in North and South America as well as the aboriginals of Australia. The results were devastating. In some places up to 95 percent of the population died quickly. Whole towns turned into massive graveyards as people caught a disease they had never encountered before. Very few were immune, so the population was intensely vulnerable.

With the disease such a devastating threat, discovering a means of stopping it became an urgent need. In a small stroke of luck, smallpox was one disease that human beings could actually figure out how to prevent using the science of the time. This search became the foundation for all modern efforts at vaccination.

VARIOLATION

Most efforts at combating smallpox were ineffective. Some physicians, following the medical practices of their time, prescribed specific herbs or beer or increased fires in a patient's room or the use of cold water. Many doctors of Elizabethan times and beyond believed that exposure to the color red would help reduce the severity of the disease. Patients were wrapped from head to toe in red cloth, and red cloth hangings were placed on beds in the sick patient's room.[15] Later scientists would argue that using red light to treat smallpox reduced scarring and decreased the course of the disease.[16] No evidence was ever found to prove this theory.

Doctors had only one procedure that not only worked to reduce the severity of smallpox but also decreased the possibility of catching it in the first place: variolation.

Variolation, also known as inoculation, is an ancient practice used in many societies where smallpox was a known scourge. Variolation is based on the principle of inducing a minor case of smallpox in order to prevent a much more severe one. The Chinese and Indians were apparently the first to practice it.[17] The idea was to take the dried scabs from smallpox survivors and use them to induce a case of smallpox in otherwise healthy people. People would inhale the smallpox pustules through their nose, come down with a milder form of the disease, and then recover. An ordinary case of wild smallpox had mortality rates of up to 30 percent.[18] Variolation had a death rate of only 1 to 2 percent.[19]

Variolation had serious drawbacks. The primary problem with this method is that it was hard to control. Health authorities of the time were not sure how much of the dried scabs were needed to induce a reaction. Sometimes the smallpox involved was very dangerous and would cause many more deaths than other variants. Using too little material ran the risk of not giving the person smallpox at all, while using too much ran the risk of causing the person to die. Using variolation could also spark another smallpox epidemic in the community after the first outbreak had run its course. No one could tell what would happen. No authorities of the day could predict who would survive and who would die. Still, many felt it was better to go through variolation than to wait for another smallpox epidemic to break out at any time.

Inoculation remained largely unknown in Europe until the 1700s. In 1717, Lady Mary Wortley Montagu went to live with her husband in Turkey, where he was the British ambassador.[20] Mrs. Montagu was keenly interested in the lives of the Turks. During her travels there she noted the Turkish practice of variolation against smallpox. As a young woman, Montagu had been stricken with the disease, with dreadful aftereffects. Smallpox took her brother's life, left her without eyelashes, and caused her to be greatly pockmarked for the rest of her life.[21] Montagu quickly realized the efficacy of the Turkish method and had her son inoculated.

Upon her return home, Montagu wrote about variolation and recommended it to her friends. She also had her daughter variolated in front of royal court doctors. In 1721 England was in the grip of yet another round of smallpox. Montagu convinced Caroline, Princess of Wales (later Queen Consort of George II), to have two of her children undergo variolation.[22] The English method differed slightly from the Turkish one. Instead of blowing dried particles into someone's nose, a puncture was made in the skin and the dried particles rubbed against it.

After the royals adopted it, inoculation became an extremely fashionable procedure. Many upper-class families insisted on variolation for all their children. However, the procedure was not popular everywhere. Clergymen denounced the method as going against God's will. In many places, people rejected it because the science was not well understood and the procedure was deemed too foreign.

Others marveled at any chance to combat smallpox. George Washington was so impressed with the method he ordered all potential revolutionary army recruits to get inoculated after an outbreak of smallpox in the colonies.[23] Frederick II of Prussia also demanded variolation for all members of his army.[24] Other rulers including Catherine the Great of Russia, Empress Maria Theresa of Austria and the reigning king of France embraced variolation for close relatives and often the general population as well.[25]

The famous American preacher Cotton Mather attempted to persuade his fellow Bostonians to use variolation after a smallpox outbreak threatened the city in 1721.[26] The campaign helped head off the worst effects but not without controversy. At one point an actual bomb was thrown at his house.

THE EDWARD JENNER STORY

Variolation was a useful stopgap. It worked somewhat effectively and reduced the spread of smallpox. People were grateful to have even some minor means of protecting themselves against a disease everyone found terrifying. Still, it was an unsatisfying method at best. The world continued to experience periodic waves of smallpox, with no predictable way to stop them or mitigate their effects.

In 1756, a young man named Edward Jenner underwent variolation. Two decades later, Jenner's efforts to find a more effective substitute for the procedure would win him fame and save countless lives.

Edward Anthony Jenner was born in the English town of Berkeley, roughly two hundred miles west of London. His father was the local reverend and a prosperous landowner. Within five years of his birth, both of his parents had died. Jenner was taken in by an older sister and given a well-rounded early education. When he was fourteen, he went off to London for a seven-year apprenticeship in medicine. Nine years later, Jenner returned to rural Berkeley to serve as the area's doctor. His knowledge of farming techniques would provide him with an excellent background for his medical experiments.

As a doctor, Jenner became well-versed in the practice of variolation and used it on his patients frequently. Unfortunately, he was also well aware of the risks it carried. Like many of his fellow doctors of the time, Jenner wanted a more effective method of protection against smallpox.

He found it on the farm.

On the farms of that time period, milkmaids were the girls and women who milked cows and then prepared dairy products. Many people had long noticed that these milkmaids rarely caught smallpox. Jenner was the first to conduct experiments to find out why. He would go on to use these results to unlock the key to the greatest medical breakthrough in history. His contribution to medicine would not only help begin the eradication of smallpox but also provide the means of protecting against many other deadly diseases.

Cows harbor a virus known as cowpox. Milkmaids would get cowpox from the cow's udders, feel a bit under the weather for a few days, and then never get it again. Cowpox also provided a huge measure of protection against smallpox. Why? Because smallpox is closely related to cowpox. The diseases are so similar that the body cannot differentiate between the two. As a result, people whose bodies create substances that protect against cowpox (called antibodies) can then use these same substances as protection against smallpox.

While Jenner became world famous for his efforts against smallpox, he was also curious about many other areas of science and medicine. Before his interest in and work with smallpox, Jenner discovered a way to reduce the toxicity of a common medication for parasitic diseases, found out that cuckoos laid their eggs in other birds' nests, and identified a cause of heart disease pain. This prior knowledge of the scientific principles of his day served him well in his quest for a smallpox vaccine.

During this time doctors often conducted experiments that would not be allowed today because they would be considered far too dangerous. Jenner took advantage of this fact with the first of his experiments on smallpox. In May 1796, a young milkmaid approached him with a clear case of cowpox. Jenner wanted to find out if he could use her obvious case of cowpox to infect someone with cowpox and thereby provide that person with possible protection against smallpox. To do this, Jenner needed another person who he could potentially infect with cowpox and who was known not to have had smallpox. Jenner found his subject in the person of his gardener's child, James Phipps. Phipps was eight at the time and had not been subject to the rigors of variolation yet. The boy's father agreed to let his son be Jenner's first test subject.

The doctor deliberately infected Phipps with cowpox by poking his arm with a few scratches and then rubbing in the cowpox material from his milkmaid in the wound. This was the normal procedure used for variolation. Where Jenner's procedure differed from normal was in using the far less dangerous cowpox as a medium instead of smallpox. The doctor then purposely tried to get the young boy to develop smallpox by exposing him to material containing smallpox pustules. Phipps remained free of any smallpox symptoms despite repeated introduction to smallpox materials.

This was the first known demonstration that people could use a mild form of one disease to provide protection against another disease. This procedure became known as inoculation. Today, the terms inoculation, vaccination, and immunization are used interchangeably, although they technically refer to slightly different procedures. Jenner's findings would soon become one of the foundations of modern medicine and form the basis for most vaccine efforts for over a century.

After he felt confident he had succeeded with one person, he tested his method on an additional twenty-three people. To his delight, not one of them came down with smallpox. His results were widely publicized after he wrote a treatise he called *An Inquiry into the Causes and Effects of the Variolae Vaccinae: A Disease Discovered in Some of the Western Counties of England, Particularly Gloucestershire, and Known by the Name of the Cow Pox.*

Some members of the medical profession were initially opposed to his methods because they felt they were dangerous and unproven, foreshadowing the current claims of the modern anti-vaccine movement. Some doctors also resented the possibility that Jenner might make their lucrative specialty of variolation obsolete. But in less than a decade, the efficacy of his techniques became clear, and public health authorities lent their official support to his discovery. Jenner's innovation was to prove that one could use cowpox, a relatively minor illness, in great quantities to help prevent smallpox, a virulently deadly disease. While he would not live to see further use of his ideas, his general principles came to be applied to many other infectious diseases.

Early vaccination could often be a dangerous affair and was at best a minor improvement on variolation. Cowpox samples were not always easy to get. The pus used could simply become contaminated with smallpox, thus rendering it ineffective and promoting an outbreak of the very disease it was supposed to prevent. But smallpox was so scary and variolation so uncertain that many people still asked for inoculation. Jenner spent the last decades of his life attempting to refine his initial methods to make them safer and easier on the patient. Jenner also gave away his vaccination to many poor children.

Jenner continued to face opposition to his vaccination efforts his entire life. As soon as he published his results, people rushed to attack him. Early vaccine opponents made many of the same arguments then that opponents make today. Vaccination was said to be ineffective or a violation of bodily integrity or even to turn people into cows.

Even after the vaccine was better developed and refined, it was still a relatively hazardous procedure for many decades. High fevers were not uncommon, as were very swollen lymph nodes. Young children and people with compromised immune systems were especially at risk from complications that could even include encephalitis. Deaths from the early vaccines were not unknown. Fortunately, modern vaccines are infinitely safer and have significantly fewer and far more minor side effects.

Luckily for British citizens, British health officials ignored the arguments against the vaccine because they saw how well it worked. They pushed laws into place designed to spread the procedure to the entire population. The UK Vaccination Act of 1840 provided free smallpox vaccination for the poor. The 1853 act went further and mandated vaccination for all children by the time they were four months old. People who did not vaccinate their children or themselves could be fined or jailed.

In other countries, Jenner's contribution was greeted with initial delight. Napoleon ordered vaccination for all his troops who had not had the disease before. Thomas Jefferson admired the procedure so much he actually learned how to perform it and personally vaccinated many people. By 1810, vaccination was declared mandatory in Bavaria, Denmark, and the Grand Duchy of Hesse.

Opposition to Jenner's smallpox vaccine would continue during his lifetime and for decades afterward. In 1853 the Anti-Vaccination League was founded in London, and in 1867 the Anti-Compulsory Vaccination League followed. The society would morph into the National Anti-Vaccination League and open offices in other countries including the United States. An 1885 anti-vaccine protest brought out more than a hundred thousand people and led to a British commission to investigate the protestors' claims. In 1896, British health authorities declared that vaccination against smallpox was ideal but allowed people to claim exemptions without fear of fine or public censure.

Between 1879 and 1885, three separate American anti-vaccine societies were formed after vaccination rates fell and smallpox receded. Health officials spent a great deal of time combating the misinformation they put out. Similar movements spread to several other countries including Belgium and Switzerland. Opposition to vaccines continues today.

In spite of objections, vaccination efforts against smallpox continued apace. By 1950, smallpox vaccination had eliminated the disease from all but four countries in the Western hemisphere. Yet more than fifty million cases continued to erupt each year. In 1958, Victor Zhdanov, a Russian virologist, started a campaign to push for the elimination of smallpox from the entire world. The World Health Organization made it a priority. On December 9, 1979, a commission of world-class scientists declared that smallpox was officially the first disease conquered by human efforts.

Those efforts would not have been possible without the existence of Jenner's vaccine.

With the end of smallpox came the end of an era. No mother today mourns the loss of her children because of this once-dreaded disease. No one faces a lifetime of blindness because of smallpox. We have no massive burials of victims; see no faces pockmarked because of an illness that once killed millions each year; no longer live with the constant threat that the "speckled monster" will periodically come into our communities and leave behind only grief.

In short, today we see the ultimate results of Jenner's experiments. Without his daring work and vehement defense of his methodology and hypothesis, smallpox might still claim the lives of millions even today.

The Biology of Vaccines

THE IMMUNE SYSTEM, OR YOUR BODY IS PRETTY DARN SMART

*V*accines are created based on a few basic principles that many of us learn in high school biology. The science is both well established and fairly well understood.

One of the essential rules of modern biology is that most of us have the same basic body parts. We have the same number of fingers and toes, the same brain structure, and the same internal organs. This has remained true for thousands of years. Strip away our skin, and biologically, we're all pretty much the same person underneath.

This is a huge stroke of luck. If I give someone an aspirin, I can be assured that one person will get mostly the same pain relief from it as any other person. Similarly, this person will likely get the same side effects, as well. This principle is one of the foundations of modern medicine.

Another huge stroke of luck is that most of us happen to have a functional immune system that works in mostly the same way from person to person. Your immune system is your body's defense against anything that appears as if it might harm your body. The immune system consists of varying types of defenses, creating an overall biological mechanism designed to protect your body against potential diseases.

The immune system aims to fight off two primary invaders: bacteria and viruses. Bacteria are microorganisms that live everywhere, including your own body. Most bacteria are harmless. In fact, most bacteria are quite necessary for our own health and even enjoyment. Without this kind of organism, we wouldn't have cheese, bread, or wine. Unfortunately, some bacteria can cause dangerous infections such as meningitis and pneumonia. Viruses, like bacteria, are microorganisms, but they are even tinier. They can also invade the body and cause diseases such as chicken pox and the flu.

Your immune system consists of interlocking cells, tissues, and specific organs that work together to make sure you don't get sick from microorganisms such as bacteria and viruses. Your immune system also helps lessen symptoms if you get sick. Our bodies essentially have three direct layers of protection against germs. The first layer is your skin. The second is a nonspecific immune response that causes redness and swelling at the site of the injury, followed by the body's attempt at healing with the production of pus and new skin.

The third kind of immune system protection is your white blood cells. Most healthy people have several kinds of white blood cells that constantly circulate in our blood and through our organs. We also have specific organs devoted to helping our immune systems function, such as the spleen. Your white blood cells have two aims: to remember invaders and to destroy them. A person in good health has a lot of white blood cells because it takes a lot of cells to kill invaders and because we're often under attack from germs.

Make no mistake. In any given day, your body encounters a storm of biological attackers. Stroll down any major city block and the air you breathe contains microscopic particles that can get into your lungs and cause serious long-term dangers. Country life offers no protection either. A single walk in a garden can produce hundreds of potential assailants. Bees, birds, plants, and virtually any living substance can easily latch onto you and start an assault on your internal organs.

Fortunately, your body's immune system is both inherently smart and primed for action. Most people's immune systems can actually tell the difference between what is part of you and what is not. The moment a potential invader enters, cells spring into action. Microbes—microscopic organisms such as viruses and bacteria—are examined closely and then attacked by millions and millions of white blood cells if deemed a threat. White cells are further divided into five specific categories. Some white cells specialize in attacking bacterial or fungal infections. A white blood cell can kill invaders in several different ways, including by releasing chemicals or even eating them.

Your white cells have a very exact and extremely useful function that vaccines utilize. This amazing property is the ability to not only recognize current threats but also remember old ones you've already battled successfully.

VACCINES WORK WITH YOUR IMMUNE SYSTEM

Vaccines take full advantage of this natural biological process. They work primarily by tapping into the memory function of your immune system. Once you get sick with certain diseases, you can never get sick from them again even if you spend hours in a room with an infected person who has a very contagious disease. If your body encounters that specific disease-causing substance again, it will immediately fight it off using the various types of white blood cells and their specific attack mechanisms. You cannot get infected again. This defense is known as natural immunity. Natural immunity is what you get after you successfully survive certain illnesses. Fortunately for all of us, most people can bypass the need to actually come down with a case of measles or mumps and get the vaccine instead. Rather than spending two weeks in bed battling a high fever, sore throat, and headache, or even ending up with permanent hearing loss, sterility, or worse, you can get a single shot or a short series of shots and have the same protection. Even if the vaccine does not entirely prevent the disease, it can trigger an increased immune response that will help reduce your symptoms.

In other words, vaccines work by creating the same biological reaction you would get from the disease without actually forcing you to get sick along the way. To achieve that goal, vaccines push the body's immune system to produce substances known as antibodies. Antibodies are proteins produced by white blood cells. Your white blood cells use antibodies to kill diseases.

A substance that can provoke an immune response is known as an antigen. An antigen can be practically anything, including egg whites, pollen, chemicals, or even dirt. The average human being is exposed to hundreds of antigens every single day beginning at birth. All of our environments are filled with them everywhere you look. You cannot go through life without being exposed to multiple antigens on any given day.

Vaccines are designed to make your immune system work for you by getting your immune system to recognize antigens without having to first fight off the diseases they can trigger. After the immune system identifies an antigen, it can develop an antibody for that antigen.

Antibodies have a drawback: they can be used to fight off only specific illnesses. An antibody for measles cannot be used by the immune system to protect against diphtheria. Your immune system stores antibodies long term and calls them up when necessary. If you have already had chicken pox and you meet someone who has a current case of chicken pox, your immune system will command chicken pox antibodies to fight off any potential new infection from the infected person. Similarly, if you have received the chicken pox vaccine and you meet someone who has a current case of chicken pox, your immune system will command the antibodies created from the vaccine to fight off any potential new infection.

The creation of antibodies by the immune system is the same process whether you have received a vaccine for a disease or have had the disease itself. The benefit of vaccines is that most vaccines consist of weakened forms of diseases, plus the addition of chemicals designed to increase your immune response and preservatives designed to keep the vaccine free of contamination. If a vaccine works, it will push your body into making antibodies after you've been vaccinated. You don't necessarily need a lot of antibodies for protection. Many vaccine-preventable illnesses are dangerous precisely because they can trick the body into producing too many antibodies and thus creating serious side effects.

An effective vaccine will contain only enough antigens to help your body create just enough antibodies so you don't get sick even if you meet someone with an infectious disease. At the same time, the vaccine will not contain enough antigens to actually cause the disease itself, sparing you the possibility of serious disease symptoms.

Most vaccines are so effective that 75 percent or more of people who receive them create antibodies after a single shot. Additional shots are recommended for two reasons. The second or third shot can create the additional exposure necessary for more people to make antibodies. Vaccine-induced immunity, like other forms of immunity, may also wear off after time. Antibody levels can drop to the point where you don't have enough protection after a few years. A booster shot can raise antibody levels to provide enough protection.

PASSIVE IMMUNITY

Vaccines are especially important for babies and newborns. Newborns and young babies have underdeveloped immune systems. When you are born, you have not yet been exposed to many disease-causing organisms. As a result, babies under six months are particularly vulnerable to many vaccine-preventable diseases. Newborns and infants can acquire a form of immunity secondhand through a mother's breast milk as well as during pregnancy. This is a form of immunity known as passive immunity. Passive immunity is a means of getting antibodies to fight off illness without being exposed to a specific illness and without receiving a vaccine. Essentially, a mother transfers her immunity to certain diseases to her fetus when it gestates in her womb and afterward to her newborn if she chooses to breastfeed.

Passive immunity can serve as a form of temporary protection against illness. However, passive immunity has several drawbacks. It is temporary and often less effective at fending off diseases. At best it can provide partial protection.

ACTIVE IMMUNITY

Active immunity results when an individual's immune system directly confronts an illness. If you get a cold, you can get active immunity against that particular cold germ, so you don't get a cold from that specific germ again. Active immunity differs from passive immunity because it is not acquired secondhand. Active immunity also differs from passive immunity because it typically lasts far longer. The process of vaccination seeks to induce active immunity that will last as long as possible. Active immunity gained through illness is often referred to as natural immunity. Natural immunity and immunity gained through vaccination all work the same way.

In some instances, natural immunity can last longer than vaccine-acquired immunity. In other instances, vaccine immunity actually provides superior results. For example, both the tetanus vaccine and the Hib vaccine (which protects against meningitis) provide most people with stronger immunity than immunity gained from coming down with a case of either illness.

TYPES OF VACCINES

One of the coolest aspects of the immune system is that it doesn't actually have to meet up with the entire virus in order to develop antibodies against it. Very often a small piece is all that's necessary to provide protection. Even better, the immune system can even be induced to react against a dead virus.

Vaccines can be divided into two forms: live attenuated and inactivated. Live vaccines contain a form of the disease that has been reduced in strength. Inactivated vaccines contain only dead forms. The two vary in use. Live attenuated vaccines are designed to reproduce once in the body but only for a very short time. The short reproduction period is enough to get an antibody response and provide immunity. Inactivated vaccines are preferred by many doctors because they often have fewer side effects than their live attenuated counterparts.

Both types of vaccines have strengths and weaknesses. Live attenuated vaccines are often easier to make for certain kinds of viruses, can be more readily controlled, and mimic the natural process of acquisition of immunity very closely in the body. As a result this kind of vaccine helps provide immunity from infection that can last as long as an individual is alive with only a single dose. The measles, mumps, and rubella (MMR) vaccine is a live attenuated vaccine.

While live attenuated vaccines are very useful, they require refrigeration to retain potency, making them difficult to store in many countries where such storage methods are harder to get. A live attenuated vaccine may not work if the virus in question undergoes mutation, nor can it be given to people who are immunocompromised, such as HIV patients.

Inactivated vaccines are created using bits and pieces of a killed virus. After the virus has been killed it can still push your immune system to create antibodies. Inactivated vaccines do not require refrigeration, nor do they mutate. This kind of vaccine can be given to populations that might not be otherwise eligible to receive them such as kidney transplant patients or HIV patients. However, inactivated vaccines sometimes do not work as well as live attenuated vaccines. Several shots might be necessary for this kind of vaccine to work rather than just one or two. The hepatitis B, polio, and pneumococcal vaccines are all examples of inactivated vaccines.

Other types of vaccines include subunit vaccines containing only very specific antigens such as certain influenza vaccines, toxoid vaccines used to fight off bacterial toxins that cause illnesses such as diphtheria, and conjugate vaccines that are safer for infants. The Hib vaccine is a conjugate vaccine that is specifically designed to work with a baby's immune system.

THE VACCINE PRODUCTION PROCESS

Edward Jenner, the doctor who made the world's first vaccine, basically gathered his vaccination material and then scratched it into the recipient's skin. The modern industrialized production of vaccines is a far longer procedure. It is also thankfully much safer than Jenner's relatively crude and often risky efforts.

The process of creating a modern vaccine is quite complex. All vaccines undergo a long period of development and testing before they are brought to market. Once the basic process of making a particular vaccine has been established, efforts are continually made to refine the process in order to improve the vaccine's safety and reduce any risk of side effects.

The creation of vaccines can vary depending on the type of vaccine in question or the company in question. However, all vaccine production follows general guidelines of safety, purity, and lack of contaminants. These guidelines are dictated by the Food and Drug Administration (FDA). In all cases of vaccine development, the focus is on the highest quality of scientific methodology and cleanliness of facilities possible. There are multiple steps involved to ensure the safety and efficacy of vaccines.

VACCINE SAFETY TESTING

Making a modern vaccine requires strict adherence to quality control methods. At every stage in the manufacturing process, the potential vaccine must be carefully supervised and controlled. Scientists and researchers handling vaccine-related material don sterilized clothing designed to minimize contact with the vaccine particles. In addition, the laboratories and manufacturing facilities must be kept sterile at all times during the process.

After the vaccine is developed, but before it can be brought to market, the manufacturer must test it carefully. Most vaccines go through three separate testing processes. During the first phase, researchers give the vaccine to a small group of healthy adult volunteers. The volunteers are tested to see if they develop an immune response and have minimal side effects. Some vaccines don't produce the desired response in humans or have too many side effects, so they are discarded during this phase.

After the first step is completed satisfactorily, the second part of testing can begin. At this point, researchers expand the testing pool to include a larger number and wider variety of people. This stage may include children as participants, especially if the vaccine is targeted toward that age group. Children are never included in any scientific research without the express written permission of their parents. The aim during this time frame is to make sure the vaccine can work on a wider scale.

Vaccines also undergo a third period of testing. The third stage of testing involves an even larger group of people. At this stage, scientists are trying to determine if the vaccine works in varied environments and on people of different ethnic backgrounds. Subjects are studied closely for several years and periodically tested to determine if they remain immune from the illness the vaccine is designed to protect against. After this phase is completed, the vaccine maker can apply to the FDA to have the vaccine introduced to the general public. The vaccine must be approved by the vaccine advisory board of the Centers for Disease Control and Prevention (CDC). The board discusses the use of the vaccine and makes recommendations about the parameters of its use. This includes the age the vaccine is given as well as the target population and the number of shots required to give maximum immunity.

Once the vaccine is distributed to the general intended audience, it is still monitored closely in several different ways. Immunization experts watch the first areas where the vaccine is distributed to see if there are any unusual reports of side effects. Experts also look to see if there are any occurrences of the disease in unexpected places and populations after the vaccine is given. They aim to see if the disease may be flaring up, despite the use of the vaccine.

Scientists and researchers also read reports from the Vaccine Adverse Event Reporting System, or VAERS, to see if there is any evidence of unusual side effects. VAERS is a public self-report system, maintained by the CDC and the FDA, that allows anyone to report suspected vaccine side effects. If any one of these areas of study presents a problem, the vaccine may be withdrawn from use and efforts made to create a safer vaccine.

HERD IMMUNITY

Vaccines have other amazing properties. A vaccine has the potential to protect not only the vaccinated but the unvaccinated as well. This property is known as herd immunity.

Herd immunity works like this. Most vaccine-preventable diseases are contagious. In order for the germ to propagate itself, it constantly needs new hosts. Many germs solve this problem by being highly adept at getting into a new body. A virus can be spread to another person by many methods, including breathing in the same air as infected persons or handling material they use, such as tissues.

If the person receiving the germ is immune to the disease it causes, the germ is stuck. It cannot reproduce itself and dies out. That's why outbreaks of diseases can come and go. A disease may find a group of highly susceptible individuals and then go from person to person. Some populations are more immune to certain diseases than others. That's because more people in one population may have already had the disease than those in another population. If a population consists of a small number of immune people, the likelihood of a disease outbreak is increased.

But not everyone in a given group of people needs to be immune, either from the disease or from a vaccine, in order to stop or prevent a disease outbreak. If a certain percentage of the population is immune, then the nonimmune people are still protected because the germs cannot get a foothold in the group. The germ then dies out. If the percentage of the group that is immune reaches the necessary level so that nonimmune people are still protected, that population is said to have herd immunity.

The percentage of immune people necessary for herd immunity varies from disease to disease. Herd immunity for measles, for example, requires at least 83 percent of any given population to be vaccinated to stop measles from spreading and protect the entire community, according to the CDC.[1] For pertussis, the percentage of vaccinated members of the community required for herd immunity is 92 percent.[2]

This means that seventeen out of one hundred people in any given population can forgo a measles vaccination and the community will remain protected from the spread of the illness. Those seventeen are not completely safe. If they move to a different community where measles rates are high, they are still at risk of contracting the illness if they come into contact with someone who has it. But as long as they remain in an area where vaccination rates are high, they have at least some measure of protection. In areas where vaccination programs remain in effect and many people are vaccinated, many vaccine-preventable illnesses will show up in few if any cases. Polio, for example, has become extremely rare in the United States because our high vaccination rates help ensure herd immunity for that disease.

Herd immunity works only for contagious diseases. Some vaccine-preventable diseases, such as tetanus, are not contagious. If your neighbors get a tetanus shot, that will not reduce your risk of getting the disease if you don't get a shot as well.

Herd immunity is a marvelous property of vaccination. It protects those who cannot receive vaccinations for legitimate medical reasons as well as anyone for whom the vaccine might not be effective.

WHAT VACCINES DON'T DO

A vaccine can do an amazing job at protecting you from an illness. If you are unvaccinated against measles, you are nearly guaranteed to get measles if you are around someone who has it. If you are vaccinated, you can hang out with the person for weeks and still probably not get sick. Even if you do get sick, a vaccine can help your immune system fight off the disease better and thus lessen the course of the illness and your potential for side effects. This is true for most other vaccine-preventable diseases as well.

What can't vaccines do? They don't provide 100 percent protection against vaccine-preventable illnesses for all people. Some people can get shot after shot and yet still not make enough antigens to protect them against the illness. Some people can get a vaccine and have it work only a little bit, so their protection is basically meaningless.

Vaccines don't increase your chances of getting other illnesses. Vaccines are not a cure for all diseases. A vaccine does not change your body's fundamental chemistry, nor does it introduce toxins into your blood.

What the process of vaccination does, and does quite effectively for most people, is reduce the risk of many serious childhood illnesses.

OTHER QUESTIONS YOU MIGHT HAVE

Making a vaccine is a complex process. Understanding why and how vaccines work fortunately is not. Basically we use vaccines to create an immune response in the body without actually forcing you to get sick. Happily for most of us this process works out quite well. We get a few shots, and then we don't get diphtheria or polio or meningitis or measles. However, a few questions may remain in your mind after reading this chapter. Here are some answers to those possible questions.

Why the Same Dose for an Adult and a Child?

On the surface this question makes sense. Why should we give the same vaccine dosage to a newborn, toddler, and adult? After all, people are advised to adjust dosages of many other medications based on factors such as age and weight.

Some vaccines, such as the flu vaccine, actually follow that principle. The dose used for kids contains less vaccine material than the dose given to adults. Many other vaccines do not.

For one thing, the amount of active material in a vaccine isn't very high to begin with. Most vaccines contain only a few milligrams of active ingredient, so not much is needed in order for the vaccine to be effective. However, the primary reason the dose usually does not differ is that vaccines aren't designed to affect the entire body. A vaccine is designed to aim for your lymph system. Once there, the vaccine wants to convince your body to make antibodies. The vaccine does not need to travel throughout your entire body to do this. Once your lymph system makes antigens, the antigens will be there if and when you need them in the future. The moment you get a potential infection, the antibody will show up, hopefully to protect you. So the amount of the dosage does not need to be changed based on age or weight.

Scientists determine how much vaccine material to use during the testing phase. Using too much can increase the risk of side effects. Using too little may not provide protection against a disease. Researchers look closely at carefully controlled studies to find out what amount should work best for most people who get the vaccine.

Why Are Vaccines Given to Babies So Early?

Another question that often arises is early vaccine use. Most babies get at least one shot before they leave the hospital and several more when they are only two months old. To many people, giving vaccines at such an early age seems counterintuitive. Why, they ask, should a baby's young immune system be exposed to illnesses before it has had the chance to fully develop?

The reason it makes sense to vaccinate babies is twofold. Babies are more vulnerable to many illnesses than are adults. An adult might not exactly enjoy a bout of measles or meningitis, but an adult, unlike a baby, is less likely to suffer serious side effects from such illnesses. Newborns are especially vulnerable to all kinds of germs because they don't have the antigens that many of us older folk do. For this reason, pediatricians often recommend keeping babies at home as much as possible prior to their first well-baby visit. During that first well-baby visit, infants receive their first dose of many important vaccines.

Younger babies can cope with the weakened virus in a vaccine more easily than they can respond to a full-fledged attack of hepatitis B or an encounter with whooping cough. The attenuated or inactivated virus in a vaccine is far gentler on a baby's system than a case of the full-blown live wild virus would be.

Why Are So Many Vaccines Given at One Time?

Babies get many vaccines in their first year. Most pediatricians recommend a series of well-baby office visits before a baby reaches his first birthday. During this time a pediatrician will examine your baby closely. The doctor wants to make sure your baby is meeting all growth milestones as well as demonstrating appropriate developmental strides.

Your doctor will also give your baby several shots during the course of each visit. A pediatrician may administer four or five immunizations in a quick motion, using very tiny needles. Understandably a parent may wonder why a pediatrician gives so many shots at once. Some people argue that shots should be spaced out instead. They insist it is better to give one shot at a time and then wait to see if the child reacts to the vaccine.

This proposal has several problems. Many shots are given during a single office visit because that is the easiest time to give them. A doctor can conveniently note your baby's growth and provide him with protection against illness in fifteen minutes. Babies can easily tolerate multiple shots at one time. The active ingredient in a vaccine is an antigen. As noted in the earlier part of this chapter, your baby will come into contact with many antigens in the course of a single day. An additional five at one time are not going to create specific problems for him. Increasing the number of pediatric visits your child gets to avoid giving him multiple shots in a single visit will not reduce his risk of side effects. Delaying only increases his chances of getting sick from a vaccine-preventable disease as well as inflates the cost of seeing the pediatrician.

Why Are Some Vaccines Given Earlier Than Others?

The standard vaccine schedule calls for the administration of certain vaccines at birth or two months, while other vaccines aren't given until the baby is over a year.

Why the disparity? Why are pediatricians giving the hepatitis B vaccine a few hours after a baby is born? In contrast, why do they wait until the baby is over a year old before giving the MMR vaccine?

The answer lies in the different natures of the diseases in question. Hepatitis B can be transmitted from mother to baby as the baby passes through the birth canal. Doctors aim to help provide babies with immediate protection against the disease if possible.

The MMR vaccine is not administered until a baby reaches her first birthday for several reasons. In the first place, most infants have some immunity against the disease from their mothers. This inherited immunity should provide temporary protection for at least the first six months of life. In the second, studies show that toddlers over fifteen months are far more likely to develop the number of antibodies necessary to fight off measles infection.[3] If you are traveling to a country with a current measles outbreak, your pediatrician may recommend giving your baby the vaccine at an earlier age just in case. In the event of a local outbreak of measles, your pediatrician may also recommend giving the MMR vaccine even if your baby isn't yet a year old.

How Do I Know If the Vaccine Worked?

Most vaccines work quite well. The MMR vaccine provides immunity for over 99 percent of all recipients after two doses given at the appropriate age.[4] Sometimes the vaccine does not work. Doctors can tell if the vaccine worked in any given patient by giving a blood test known as a titer. A titer can measure your body's ability to make antibodies. If you have enough antibodies for a specific disease, you will be immune to it.

Titers are sometimes used to determine if someone has acquired immunity to a disease before undergoing medical treatment or in the event of an outbreak of a vaccine-preventable disease. Many women who are trying to conceive a child are urged to find out if they are immune to rubella. Rubella can gravely harm a fetus. If the woman is not immune, doctors suggest an MMR shot and then waiting a month before trying to get pregnant.

Why Are Some Vaccines Bundled Together?

Some vaccines are given as single shots while others are given together. Immunologists prefer to give people vaccines that have been bundled together for several reasons. Using more than one vaccine in a shot lowers costs, reduces the need to store separate vaccines, and reduces the number of shots a baby has to get. Some vaccines require special manufacturing conditions, so they are given separately. Researchers are working on methods to increase the number of vaccines in each shot to reduce the overall number of shots babies must receive.

Of Bananas and Formaldehyde, or What the Heck *Is* in Them?

Aluminum hydroxyphosphate sulfate.
2-phenoxyethanol.
Polymyxin B.

$\mathcal{O}$h my.

When you first read a list of what actually goes into vaccines, your first reaction is often somewhere between "What the heck?" and "You've *got* to be kidding me."

The names of vaccine ingredients can appear quite scary, even shocking and dismaying. Glance at any record of vaccine ingredients and you'll encounter substances that look as if they've been concocted by a group of mad scientists. A thorough scrutiny may lead to thoughts such as "What the heck is formalin? Or glutaraldehyde? And why would anyone in their right mind add formaldehyde to something you give to a baby?"

Such questions are understandable.

However, once you become acquainted with a few terms and concepts, vaccine ingredients can easily be deciphered and demystified. After reading this chapter, you will be able to understand exactly what goes into a typical MMR (measles, mumps, and rubella) or DTaP (diphtheria, tetanus, and pertussis) shot and why these particular ingredients are necessary for the vaccines to work effectively.

Just about every single vaccine contains between five and ten ingredients. Some ingredients such as water and salt need no introduction. The purpose of other, lesser known elements may not be immediately clear. A package insert with a detailed list of ingredients can be highly intimidating. This is true especially if, like most people, your last science class was in high school and you have not picked up a chemistry textbook since then. Vaccine components often have unfamiliar syllables, oddly placed numbers, and prefixes that can seem like something out of a science fiction novel.

Even someone with good knowledge of chemistry or biology may feel slightly taken aback when scanning a list of the chemicals used in many inoculations.

Your initial instinct may be to head to the Internet for answers. A five-second search can lead to scary websites arguing that vaccines are filled with bits and pieces that will, at the very least, induce a serious case of major league ouch in just about anyone. Such sites are devoted to campaigns against vaccines. These go further and actively argue that ingredients found in nearly all vaccines can cause serious side effects in a large segment of the population, ranging from high fevers to comas and, yes, even death. After reading these sites, a reasonable person might easily think sodium chloride is another word for anthrax.

Fortunately for those of us who prefer not to see our children's ribs cracked from a bout of whooping cough, or watch them spend two weeks frantically scratching from chicken pox lesions in very unpleasant places, those claims are wrong.

Scores of vaccine components are also used in many other products found in daily life. These include commonly packaged foods, familiar medications such as pills and antacids, and other household items. Indeed most ingredients used in vaccines are probably somewhere in your house right now, in the food in your cupboards, or in the soap in your shower.

Understanding exactly what vaccine ingredients do and why they are used can help calm any feelings of fear you may have as well as provide insights into a fascinating and historically important scientific process. Scientists have been experimenting with the creation of vaccines for centuries. This ongoing process is constantly being improved upon and refined.

SO, UM, WHAT'S IN THEM AGAIN?

A list of exact components for each and every vaccine currently made can be found in many different places. Your pediatrician's office can provide you with a list of each vaccine your infant will receive during a well-baby visit. Vaccine manufacturers also list what's in each vaccine they make. While the thought of contacting Pfizer or Merck directly may sound rather intimidating, many companies welcome inquiries from concerned citizens. A representative should be able to answer any questions you might have.

Another excellent place to find a list of ingredients used in each vaccine is the Centers for Disease Control and Prevention's website. The CDC has a very useful link you can click on that will tell you what's in each vaccine. You can examine the data by each vaccine or via a comprehensive list of all vaccine ingredients used in all currently manufactured vaccines.

Vaccine ingredients can be divided into five fundamental categories. An understanding of these categories is essential in order to understand what goes into every single vaccine.

- *Antigens* are used to provoke an immune reaction from the body and thus create the basis for immunity against an illness. In the course of a typical day the average baby and grown-up will be exposed to many different antigens. A baby may pick up an object from the floor when you're not looking or sniff a flower and thus come into contact with an antigen. Antigens found in vaccines include killed viruses, weakened live viruses, and specific pieces of viruses that can still provoke an immune response and make someone safe from a disease. Antigens are also found in the human body naturally.
- *Fluids* are used to provide a medium for the rest of the ingredients in the vaccines. Most vaccines use sterilized water as a medium.
- *Preservatives and stabilizers* help make sure the vaccine remains safe for use for an extended period of time. While many parents understandably prefer to avoid preservatives, such chemicals are vital in the production of vaccines. Without the use of these chemicals, many vaccines would have a very short shelf life. Vaccines would not last as long and would become far more costly to manufacture. Babies and children who receive vaccines that have not been preserved properly can easily become sick from spoiled vaccines. Preservatives act as an insurance policy and remain essential even in communities and countries with easy access to safe storage facilities. In developing nations, preservatives help make vaccines affordable to far more people. Commonly used preservatives in vaccines are benign substances that include gelatin, monosodium glutamate (also called MSG), and glycine.
- *Adjuvants* are chemicals used to help a vaccine work more effectively. Adjuvants can help your body react more strongly to the vaccine and thus provoke a stronger immune reaction and better overall protection from the actual disease. They also often allow manufacturers to use less actual disease virus or bacteria in the vaccine. This reduces the risk of side effects from the disease antigen. Examples of adjuvants include aluminum salts.

- *Growing medium*, while not an active component of the vaccine, sometimes "comes along for the ride" when antigens are added. Growing
medium is simply the material in which the antigens were cultivated.
Chicken egg protein is a common growing material. That's why people with severe egg allergies sometimes can't receive certain vaccines.

A BIT OF MATH FIRST, OR WHY PARACELSUS GOT IT RIGHT

To truly understand what's in vaccines, a little understanding of math is necessary. Vaccine amounts are measured in very, very, very, very small doses. A
standard vaccine will include quantities no larger than a few drops of water.
Much of what goes into vaccines often requires either really superhuman
eyesight or a microscope to actually see it up close.

Philippus Aureolus Theophrastus Bombastus von Hohenheim was
a man of many interests including philosophy, chemistry, medicine, and
astronomy. Von Hohenheim is more widely known by the name he took
later in life: Paracelsus. Paracelsus was originally from what is present-day
Switzerland. When not teaching university students, dabbling in medicine,
or creating the modern forerunner of the study of botany, he made one of the
most accurate statements uttered about the subject of chemistry: "All things
are poison, and nothing is without poison; only the dose permits something
not to be poisonous."[1] In other words, the dose makes the poison.

In this single sentence, he summed up the one essential principle behind
all vaccine ingredients.

Anything at all in the entire world can either act as a poison or be utterly and completely harmless depending upon the quantity involved. And by
anything we mean literally anything. Drink too much water—an ingredient
vital for survival—and you will drown. Take too much vitamin A and you
will poison yourself. Even chocolate (alas!) can be very harmful should you
celebrate Valentine's Day with just a little too much glee.

The same is true in reverse. Anything ever measured will not harm you
in small enough quantities. Arsenic was widely used historically as a poison
and at the same time as a medicine. A handful of molecules of arsenic will
pass through your system unnoticed. A few microns of lead will not give your
child lead poisoning.

This principle is vital for understanding how vaccine ingredients are used.
Many of the substances found in vaccines, such as hydrochloric acid, we may
think unsafe. Indeed they can be. Drink an entire class of hydrochloric acid and
you will not be happy with the results. However this principle again depends on
the quantity in question. The small amount of hydrochloric acid in all vaccines
has no more effect on the human body than a glass of orange juice.

SO HOW MUCH IS THAT EXACTLY?

Now you have a list of vaccine ingredient categories. You may be wondering exactly how much material we're discussing here.

Most vaccines are measured in dosages of milliliters. A liter is a unit of measurement for fluids. One liter is roughly equivalent to a quart of liquid, or the amount in four cups of water. A milliliter (abbreviated ml) is one-thousandth of a liter, which is roughly equal to one-fifth of a teaspoon of liquid.

The active ingredients in most vaccines make up about half of a milliliter, or one-tenth of a teaspoon, or about half a drop of water.

Vaccine ingredients are further broken down into even smaller amounts. Most vaccines are actually primarily composed of plain filtered water.

Some of the materials used in vaccines aren't liquid. Some are solids that dissolve in the liquid, like adding a spoonful of sugar to a cup of coffee. Solids in vaccines are measured by weight in grams. A gram is roughly equivalent in weight to a thumbtack—in other words, a relatively small amount of material. For example, an American penny weighs two and a half grams. A typical solid material in vaccines is measured in terms of milligrams and micrograms. A milligram (abbreviated mg) is one-thousandth of a gram, or roughly the weight of a grain of sand. An even smaller and equally common measurement used in vaccines is the microgram. A microgram is one-thousandth of a milligram. A microgram (abbreviated mcg) very often cannot be seen with the naked eye.

Different manufacturers may vary the ingredients in each vaccine slightly. For example, one manufacturer may add a marginally different amount of a substance to its version of the hepatitis B vaccine. Another manufacturer may add different ingredients to that kind of vaccine. However, nearly all vaccines for a specific disease will have the same basic components in the vaccine. One manufacturer's DTaP vaccine will contain roughly the same ingredients in the same amount as another's.

COMMON INGREDIENTS FOUND
IN VACCINES AND WHAT THEY DO

Let's get specific and look at some actual vaccine ingredients.

A full list of vaccine ingredients would span several pages and include chemicals that are found in only a handful of vaccines. We have largely left them out because thankfully relatively few of us will need a rabies shot or an inoculation designed to protect us against typhoid or yellow fever. Many common vaccines utilize similar ingredients because they are known to be effective.

More common vaccine ingredients may seem initially unfamiliar or even terrifying but are actually found in many products on the supermarket shelves and even in foods you may eat several times a week. Even the popular cosmetic treatment Botox contains many of the same ingredients as vaccines.

For example, formaldehyde is undeniably added to certain vaccines. However, formaldehyde is also created in the human body as a result of normal biological functions. Indeed, it is required for the creation of amino acids, the building blocks of protein. The amount of formaldehyde found in a vaccine is comparable to the amount found in a normal human being on a typical day. Yes, a list of ingredients of the average human being would actually include formaldehyde.

In other words the average person, just like the average vaccine, contains materials that are considered toxins in certain circumstances.

Forms of aluminum are added to certain vaccines in order to help increase the body's reaction to the vaccine. Yes, aluminum is a known neurotoxin. But not in the quantities found in a typical vaccine. According to the Agency for Toxic Substances and Disease Registry, a typical adult consumes between seven and nine milligrams of aluminum every single day just by breathing and eating many common foods.[2] An average vaccine contains a far smaller amount of aluminum. Your baby will get roughly four milligrams of aluminum from his first six months of shots.[3] This is comparable to the amount found in about forty ounces of infant formula.[4] Aluminum is the world's third most common element and can also be found in many foods including dry cake mixes, tea leaves, and even breast milk.[5]

By the time a child is six, she will have most likely received fifteen vaccines containing aluminum. Meanwhile, given the amount of aluminum in breast milk, that very same child will have ingested the very same amount of aluminum from breast milk in a single year of standard nursing.

Here's a list of common vaccine ingredients and exactly what purpose they serve.

Albumin

Albumin is a simple protein found in many mammals including humans, chickens, and cows. It is often derived from eggs. Albumin is used as a culture medium to grow cells. This substance is used in several types of vaccines including the MMR, chicken pox, and flu vaccines. The amount of albumin contained in such vaccines is roughly several micrograms, much less than the amount in a standard egg.[6]

Aluminum Hydroxide, Aluminum Hydroxyphosphate Sulfate

Aluminum hydroxide and aluminum hydroxyphosphate sulfate are chemical compounds of similar composition. They are used as an adjuvant, a substance that helps increase the efficacy of the vaccine. Aluminum hydroxide is used in a number of vaccines including types of the DTaP and hepatitis B vaccines. It is also used in other medications, including antacids to reduce the effects of excess stomach acid and neutralize heartburn. The amount of aluminum hydroxide found in the Pediarix, or five-in-one vaccine (diphtheria, pertussis, tetanus, polio, and hepatitis B), is 0.625 milligrams.[7] In comparison, infant formula contains 0.225 milligrams of aluminum per liter.[8]

Aluminum hydroxyphosphate sulfate can be found in types of the Hib, hepatitis A, and hepatitis B vaccines as well as Gardasil, the cervical cancer vaccine. The Gardasil vaccine contains 0.225 milligrams of this chemical, or the same amount found in a quart of infant formula.[9]

Studies have found no difference in neurological events between children given vaccines containing aluminum and children given vaccines without aluminum.[10]

Amino Acids

Amino acids are chemicals that serve as the building blocks for proteins. Such chemicals play a vital role in important life processes such as nutrition. Amino acids such as glycine are used in vaccines as a stabilizer. Commonly used vaccines where amino acids may be found include forms of the hepatitis B vaccine.

Formaldehyde, Formalin

Formaldehyde is a naturally occurring organic compound. When dissolved in water, formaldehyde is referred to as formalin. Formaldehyde has several uses in vaccines. The compound is used to inhibit the growth of potentially harmful bacteria, inactivate toxins in certain specific vaccines, and help preserve the vaccine's efficacy. When ingested or inhaled in larger quantities, formaldehyde and formalin can indeed have very harmful effects. However, in the quantities used in vaccines, both substances are harmless. Your own body produces and excretes minute quantities of formaldehyde every time you digest food.

Formaldehyde is also found naturally in many foods including apricots, pears, potatoes, shrimp, and coffee.[11] Formaldehyde can be found in many vaccines including types of the DTaP, hepatitis B, Hib, and polio vaccines.[12]

All vaccines combined contain roughly 1.2 milligrams of formaldehyde. In contrast a kilogram of bananas (about three whole medium-sized bananas) contains 16.3 milligrams of naturally occurring formaldehyde.[13]

Feed your baby a single mashed banana, and he'll get more formaldehyde from that piece of fruit than from every vaccine on the standard vaccine schedule combined.

Gelatin

Gelatin is a protein derived from collagen and commonly used in many foodstuffs including Jell-O, jams, marshmallows, and yogurt as well as in cosmetics, photography, and medication production. Gelatin is used in vaccines as a stabilizer. Common vaccines that contain gelatin include types of the DTaP, hepatitis B, MMR, and varicella, or chicken pox, vaccines.[14]

Glutaraldehyde

Glutaraldehyde is an organic compound. Very tiny amounts of glutaraldehyde are used in vaccines as a toxin detoxifier. Other applications for glutaraldehyde (in much higher concentrations) include as a fertilizer for aquatic plants and as a disinfectant for medical equipment. Roughly fifty nanograms, or one-billionth of a gram, of glutaraldehyde can be found in the stand-alone DTaP vaccine and the five-in-one Pediarix vaccine.[15,16]

Hydrochloric Acid

Hydrochloric acid is a compound of hydrogen and chlorine. When consumed directly, it can cause great harm. However, hydrochloric acid is also a widely occurring substance found in many places, including your stomach where it is secreted naturally. Hydrochloric acid is used to adjust a vaccine's pH, or the acidity of a substance. Some vaccines may have problems with alkalinity once all ingredients have been added, so a minute addition of hydrochloric acid is necessary in order to bring the entire vaccine into the right pH. Without this ingredient the vaccine might actually trigger a strong reaction that could be very dangerous.

Hydrochloric acid can be found in types of the DTaP vaccine.[17]

Killed Viruses

Viruses are infectious agents that can reproduce only in the cells of living creatures. People create an immune response when infected with a live virus, making us more resistant in the future to an illness. Killed viruses can serve the same purpose but with greatly reduced risks. A killed virus is used in certain vaccines to create an immune response. The body will still produce a reaction even when the virus has died. Killed viruses are used in some polio and flu vaccines.[18]

Monosodium Glutamate

Also known by the initials *MSG*, monosodium glutamate is a form of salt often added as a flavor enhancer to certain foods. It is added to vaccines in order to help preserve their long-term efficacy. Forms of the flu, MMR, and chicken pox vaccines contain amounts of MSG.[19] The FluMist vaccine contains 0.188 milligrams of MSG.[20] By contrast, grape juice contains 0.258 milligrams of MSG per 100 grams.[21] Peas contain 0.200 milligrams of MSG per 100 grams.[22] Even human breast milk contains 0.22 milligrams of naturally occurring MSG per 100 grams.[23]

Neomycin

Neomycin is a common antibiotic that can be used on the skin or taken orally. It is used in vaccines to inhibit the growth of bacteria. Treating the average infection typically requires between twenty and forty milligrams of neomycin per kilogram of body weight per day.[24] A vaccine typically contains less than one milligram in total of neomycin. Common vaccines that contain neomycin include types of the MMR, polio, and chicken pox vaccines.[25]

Partial Bacteria

Bacteria are a type of microscopic living organism that can be found all over the world including in soils and inside human beings. Bits of bacteria can be used to provoke an immune response that helps ward off infection. Vaccines that are made from partial bacteria include forms of the Hib and DTaP.[26]

Partial Viruses

A virus is a form of infectious agent that is capable of replication only within the cells of a living creature. Parts of certain viruses are used in vaccines in order to generate an immune response that will protect the person against the disease in question. The entire virus is not needed to create this response. Vaccines that use partial viruses include forms of the hepatitis B and Gardasil vaccines.[27]

Phenoxyethanol, 2-Phenoxyethanol

Phenoxyethanol and 2-phenoxyethanol are different names for the same organic chemical compound. Phenoxyethanol can be found in many household items including perfumes, sunscreen, and cosmetics. It is used in vaccines as a preservative. Many childhood vaccines contain this chemical including the Pediarix, DTaP, hepatitis B, and polio vaccines.[28] The DTaP vaccine contains 2.5 milligrams of phenoxyethanol.[29]

Phosphate Buffers

A phosphate buffer is a solution designed to help a chemical maintain a constant pH level. Making sure a substance is neither too alkaline nor too acidic can help reduce the chances the vaccine will trigger an unwanted reaction and increase the chances the vaccine will work more effectively. Examples of phosphate buffers used in vaccines include potassium (a necessary ingredient for proper organ function and found in many foods) and potassium and sodium dihydrogen phosphates (frequently used as gentle laxatives). Phosphate buffers can be found in most vaccines including types of the DTaP, flu, and chicken pox vaccines.[30]

Polymyxin B

Polymyxin B is another commonly used antibiotic that is often taken orally to treat bacterial infections. It is used in vaccines to help reduce the growth of bacteria. One-tenth of a nanogram (a billionth of a gram) can be found in the five-in-one vaccine (Pediarix) containing the DTaP, polio, and hepatitis B vaccines.[31] Similar quantities can be found as well in forms of the chicken pox, flu, and polio vaccines.[32]

Polysorbate 80

Polysorbate 80 is an additive made from glucose or a form of sugar and oleic acid, a form of fat found naturally in many animal and plant products and considered highly safe for human consumption. This additive is used in many foods and medications as well as vaccines. Polysorbate 80 acts as an emulsifier and solubilizer. Emulsifiers are used to help keep ingredients together that might normally separate, such as oil and water. Solubilizers help ingredients remain dissolved. Polysorbate 80 can be found in items such as pickles, condiments, shortening, and whipped dessert toppings as well as vitamins and liquid soaps and even ice cream, where it is used to help prevent melting. Polysorbate 80 is used in several common vaccines including kinds of the DTaP, Pediarix, Gardasil, and flu vaccines.[33]

Sodium Chloride

Sodium chloride is more commonly known as table salt. It can be found in many food items as well as inside the body, where a certain amount is necessary in order for the body's organs to function properly. Table salt is added to vaccines to help keep them in a state that will not adversely affect the cells. Most vaccines contain some form of sodium chloride.

Sorbitol

Sorbitol is a sweetener often used in place of sugar. It can be found in foods such as sugar-free chewing gum and diet drinks as well as mouthwash and cosmetics. A single stick of sorbitol-sweetened chewing gum contains approximately 1.25 grams of the substance. Sorbitol can also be found naturally in many fruits and berries. Sorbitol is added to vaccines such as the MMR as a preservative.[34]

Sucrose

Sucrose is more commonly known as sugar. Sugar is a very common ingredient that many people consume every single day. One can find sucrose used as a sweetener in prepared desserts as well as naturally in many fruits. Sucrose is added to vaccines in order to help the vaccine remain potent even when exposed to light or heat from outside sources. Sucrose is found in several vaccines including forms of the Hib, MMR, and chicken pox vaccines.[35]

Weak Live Viruses

A virus is an infectious agent that can reproduce only inside a living cell. During the manufacturing process for some vaccines, live viruses are weakened so they can no longer do any harm to the body. A weakened virus can be strong enough to provoke an immune response that will protect someone against the disease yet cause no harm. Weakened live viruses are used in certain vaccines including forms of the MMR and chicken pox vaccines.[36]

Yeast Protein

Yeast is one of the culture media used to grow the cells necessary to create vaccines. Very small quantities remain in certain vaccines after the vaccines have been removed from the culture. Vaccines that contain yeast protein include Pediarix and types of the hepatitis B and Hib vaccines.[37]

PUTTING IT ALL TOGETHER:
THE MMR VACCINE EXAMINED CLOSE UP

Now that we've gone through a list of vaccine ingredients, let's put them all together and look more closely at a specific vaccination.

One of the most important childhood vaccines is the MMR vaccine. Measles is a very contagious illness with side effects that include high fever and hearing loss. A case of the mumps can lead to painful swelling in a little boy's testicles and infertility later in life. Rubella, while often harmless in older children and adults, can cause mental retardation, blindness, and deafness in a fetus.

The entire MMR vaccine contains approximately half a milliliter of fluid (half a drop of liquid), most of it in the form of water. The vaccine consists entirely of the following components:

- live attenuated measles virus
- live attenuated mumps virus
- live attenuated rubella virus
- sorbitol
- sodium phosphate
- sucrose
- sodium chloride
- hydrolyzed gelatin
- human serum albumin
- fetal bovine serum
- neomycin
- residual egg proteins
- chicken-embryo cell culture
- human-diploid WI-38 cell culture

The measles, mumps, and rubella viruses are used as antigens to trigger the body's immune response. The levels of these viruses in the MMR vaccine can be measured in micrograms. Sorbitol (14.5 micrograms) is a form of sugar used to help stabilize the vaccine ingredients.[38] Sodium phosphate and/or sucrose (1.9 milligrams) is used to help control the pH level. Sodium chloride and hydrolyzed gelatin combined add up to 14.5 milligrams in the MMR vaccine.[39] Sodium chloride also helps to control the pH level of the vaccine. Gelatin acts as a stabilizer. Human serum albumin (0.3 milligrams) is a protein found in human blood plasma and used as a culture medium to grow cells necessary to create the vaccine. Fetal bovine serum is an additional culture medium. Neomycin (25 micrograms) is an antibiotic added to the

MMR vaccine to help reduce bacterial growth.[40] The two cell cultures at the end of the list are growth mediums.

In short, the MMR vaccine contains very small amounts of each material. Each individual part is used in quantities that can barely be measured and are harmless when injected as a whole.

A CLOSER LOOK AT YOUR LOCAL TUNA FISH SANDWICH

A simple comparison can help put individual vaccine ingredients in perspective. A standard tuna fish sandwich is usually made from white bread, canned tuna, mayonnaise, and a bit of chopped celery and onions.

Just as a look at vaccine ingredients can appear quite creepy upon immediate reading, so too can a quick look at the list of ingredients on the side of a commonly purchased package of white bread.

A loaf of Wonder bread contains enriched wheat flour, water, salt, and wheat gluten.[41]

It may also contain some of the following ingredients:

- ferrous sulfate
- soy fiber
- cottonseed fiber
- sodium stearoyl lactylate
- ethoxylated mono- and diglycerides
- mono- and diglycerides
- datem
- calcium dioxide
- dicalcium phosphate
- cellulose gum
- calcium carbonate
- ammonium sulfate
- monocalcium phosphate
- ammonium phosphate
- ammonium chloride
- calcium sulfate
- calcium propionate[42]

Many such ingredients don't exactly leap off the tongue or even appear to have much to do with bread. Yet at the same time such ingredients are often used for benevolent purposes that help the bread in question last longer and taste better without being harmful to public health.

Ferrous sulfate is a form of iron deliberately added to help the general public avoid medical conditions such as anemia that can stem from a lack of iron. Sodium stearoyl lactylate is a chemical compound made from salt, lactic acid, and sodium hydroxide. The compound acts as an emulsifier, or a substance that helps ingredients remain mixed together. Sodium stearoyl lactylate can help dough retain moisture and disperse fats evenly. Ammonium chloride helps yeast grow.

Canned tuna also contains some ingredients that can seem quite frightening at first. A typical can of tuna may contain pyrophosphate, hydrolyzed protein, and even methylmercury.[43] Pyrophosphates help cells function better. Methylmercury is a form of mercury that can have dangerous side effects, but quantities in tuna are limited to less than one part per million, a level that has been declared safe by the Food and Drug Administration (FDA).[44]

Most tuna fish sandwiches contain mayonnaise. Homemade mayonnaise is usually a mixture of oil, egg, and vinegar. Most commercial mayonnaises contain salt, sugar, mustard, lemon juice, and an additive known as EDTA. EDTA (an abbreviation for ethylenediaminetetraacetic acid) is a chemical compound used to preserve food freshness. EDTA is employed in certain medicinal processes such as chelation therapy as a way to help remove excess dangerous heavy metals from the blood. EDTA is also used in two vaccines: the rabies vaccine and the chicken pox vaccine.[45]

Even a seemingly harmless ingredient such as celery contains pesticide residue. The nonprofit public health organization Environmental Working Group placed celery second on its list of most contaminated fruit and vegetables.[46] When washed, minute amounts of pesticides (in quantities measured in micrograms) still remain.

Our point here is not to urge people away from eating tuna fish sandwiches. Tuna is an excellent source of protein with many potential benefits. But tuna fish sandwiches, like vaccines, can superficially appear to contain poisons. Many ordinary foods that people willfully consume contain very small amounts of chemicals that sound terrifying yet pose no danger when consumed in such small amounts.

WHAT'S *NOT* IN VACCINES

Vaccines do indeed contain some undeniably scary ingredients.

Some anti-vaccine groups go even further. They allege that vaccines contain material they don't. For example, a common assertion by many vaccine critics is that vaccines contain antifreeze.

Yikes.

Um, no, not really. Not even close.

Antifreeze is actually a very useful material that allows modern society to function better. A chemical compound composed of various substances, it is used to raise the boiling point of water and lower the freezing point. This helps make engines work more smoothly and thus lets your car run better when it's very cold outside. Antifreeze is also used to help prevent plane crashes in bad weather.

Using antifreeze can have problems. Many forms of antifreeze have a sweet taste to them. A dog or child that laps up even a small quantity can die from the effects. The material can also be toxic to the environment, so you may have to bring in large amounts to a center with the right facilities to dispose of it properly.

In other words, antifreeze is toxic stuff that has to be handled carefully. Antifreeze is not used in anything people eat because it's not safe to consume. This includes vaccines.

Some vaccines (as we've pointed out) do indeed contain a substance known as 2-phenoxyethanol or phenoxyethanol. Phenoxyethanol contains propylene glycol.

Antifreeze contains a substance known as ethylene glycol. While both antifreeze and phenoxyethanol have the word *glycol* as a component, the two forms are not even remotely the same. Ethylene glycol can turn into oxalic acid when ingested and damage the heart, kidneys, and central nervous system in large enough amounts. Propylene glycol is a type of mineral oil widely used in many different products. Propylene glycol is consumed by many people on a daily basis because it is added to certain foods and beverages including soda, cookies, ice cream, and salad dressing. You've probably harmlessly ingested at least a bit of it in the last few months.

Another common ingredient that some vaccine critics claim is found in vaccines is aborted fetal tissue.

Is this true?

Well, no, but . . .

This one is a bit more complicated.

No vaccine contains aborted fetal tissue. However, during the vaccine creation process the viruses used to make certain vaccines such as the MMR are cultured from media that contain human fetal cells.

In other words, the vaccine does not contain such tissue, but the process used to create the vaccine relies on such tissue. The culture media derive from cells obtained from two legally aborted fetuses from the 1960s. These media have been used ever since to culture vaccines. They have also been used in many other types of medical research designed to study aspects of human biology and microbiology.

The Catholic Church's stance against abortion is widely known. Officials from the church have weighed on the matter of vaccines with an official policy statement. In a 2005 statement from the Vatican Pontifical Academy for Life, church officials argued that although it was wrong in a sense to make vaccines from such cells, it is acceptable practice for people to use such vaccines today. The church stated that usage was acceptable because vaccines undeniably save lives. Officials further stated that "in a particular context such as that in the United States, it is licit to use these vaccines, because there are no others actually available."[47]

In summary the ingredients found in vaccines are not harmful in the quantities used. Once you learn the terminology, it is easy to understand exactly why. Chemicals and materials mistakenly labeled as toxins are everywhere including in the air you breathe, the food you eat, and the water you drink. It is impossible to go about modern life without encountering them. Human beings have developed multiple ways to cope with this fact and even take advantage of it. Our bodies are designed to ingest such minute amounts of chemicals and extract use from them. Our bodies are equally designed to then excrete chemicals via internal organs. This is what your kidneys and liver are for.

These principles apply equally to newborns, infants, toddlers, children, and adults.

THIMEROSAL SHIMEROSAL, OR WHY ETHYLMERCURY AND METHYLMERCURY ARE NOT THE SAME THING

Perhaps the most controversial ingredient ever added to vaccines at any point in time is a substance known as thimerosal.

Thimerosal is an organic compound that contains a small amount of mercury. A compound is a chemical substance that contains at least two elements. Compounds can be broken into distinct elements by means of a chemical reaction. An organic compound is a compound that contains carbon.

Thimerosal was added to vaccines in order to kill potentially deadly bacteria and to act as a preservative. Preservatives are necessary to help make sure that vaccines can remain in use for a longer period of time. Without the use of such preservatives vaccines would have a much shorter shelf life. The costs of manufacturing vaccines would increase, and more people would risk serious illness as a result of contaminated vaccines.

In addition to vaccines, thimerosal has also been added to various medical and cosmetic products since the 1920s, including nasal sprays and contact lens cleaning products. The preservative was and is used only in vaccines that do not contain live viruses because its usage would have rendered the vaccines ineffective. Certain vaccines, such as the MMR, have never contained thimerosal.

In the late 1990s, some members of the parenting community began to voice concerns that the addition of this chemical to vaccines was causing serious problems in children. Some parents in particular alleged that their children were developing abnormally, and such abnormal development was directly related to the administration of vaccines. Parents took a look at the list of vaccine ingredients and declared thimerosal the essential cause of their children's problems.

In 2001, a group of parents published a paper in the journal *Medical Hypotheses*. The journal is nonpeer reviewed, meaning that medical professionals and scientists do not review submissions for accuracy or scientific validity. The article was titled "Autism: A Novel Form of Mercury Poisoning." Essentially the group argued that (a) their children were suffering from autism, (b) the autism in question was from a form of mercury poisoning, and (c) thimerosal was the culprit.

On the surface, the case they made against thimerosal appears to have great merit. Autism rates appeared to be rising at the time. Some of the symptoms in question did correlate with possible mercury poisoning.

Look closer, however, and the argument they made falls apart. Symptoms of mercury poisoning include small head circumference, whereas children with autism typically have heads that are larger than normal.[48] Many people suffering from mercury poisoning have problems with muscle coordination. By contrast, the most typical motor symptoms of autism are repetitive behaviors that require muscle coordination such as rocking back and forth. Mercury poisoning also leads to vision problems. Vision problems are much less common in children with autism.[49]

The authors were right in that thimerosal is indeed a mercury compound. Mercury is not a good thing for the body. For years, scientists have classified mercury as a known neurotoxin, or a poisonous substance that harms nerve cells. The bad effects of mercury on human beings have been widely documented for centuries. The very expression "mad hatter" comes from the fact that those employed in the making of hats came into heavy contact with mercury and often became mentally ill as a result.

At the same time, accuracy demands that one distinguish between forms of a substance. Mercury exists in several different forms: inorganic mercury compounds, metallic or elemental mercury, and organic mercury compounds.

Inorganic mercury compounds are formed when mercury combines with elements such as chlorine rather than carbon. Inorganic mercury compounds can be found in items such as skin lightening creams. Elemental mercury is a heavy metal with a silvery sheen. Elemental mercury is in liquid form when at room temperature and is used in items such as thermometers and batteries. Organic mercury compounds are a mixture of carbon mercury. Organic mercury compounds come in several different forms.

Methylmercury is an organic form of mercury that has been repeatedly proven to be very dangerous to all living things. Ingestion of methylmercury can cause problems that include birth defects, a decrease in cognitive functioning, and possibly blindness and deafness.

Methylmercury is not now nor ever has been used in vaccines. However, it is the type of mercury commonly found in contaminated foods, such as fish. The type of mercury in our tuna fish sandwich is methylmercury in tiny doses.

Thimerosal consists of a form of mercury known as ethylmercury. Ethylmercury has both carbon atoms and mercury atoms.

Ethylmercury and methylmercury are not the same thing. Methylmercury is the most easily absorbed form of mercury. It can cross the blood brain barrier relatively easily. Ethylmercury is a much larger molecule and has a far less chance of getting through to the brain. It is also far more rapidly excreted from the body than methylmercury. A study in the February 1, 2008, issue of *Pediatrics*, the official journal of the American Academy of Pediatrics, found that "the blood half-life of intramuscular ethyl mercury from thimerosal in vaccines in infants is substantially shorter than that of oral methyl mercury in adults."[50] The study concluded that "a new risk assessment regarding exposure to thimerosal used as a preservative should be conducted in light of the demonstrated short half-life of ethyl mercury after vaccination."[51]

In the 1990s, the amount of thimerosal in the cumulative dosage of all vaccines on the standard vaccine schedule did exceed Environmental Protection Agency standards. It should be noted that the amount in question did not exceed World Health Organization standards or standards set by the Food and Drug Administration (FDA). As a result of concerns about the cumulative dosage, by 2002 thimerosal had been removed from nearly all vaccines. Officials did so on the basis of the precautionary principle. The precautionary principle is the notion that even if an activity has not been conclusively proven harmful, that activity should be stopped if there are possible threats to human health.

In applying this principle to the thimerosal issue, officials acted under the idea that even if thimerosal could not be proven to harm babies, there was potential for harm. Many opponents of thimerosal argued that once it was removed, one should see a drop in the number of autism cases.

The expected drop never happened.

In short, thimerosal appears to be similar to other chemicals and toxins found in vaccines. On the surface it sounds scary. Looked at more closely, the questions raised disappear.

A Real Mother:
The World Before Vaccines

$\mathcal{O}$n December 14, 1878, a sadly common tragedy played out in the halls of a castle in a small corner of Germany. Queen Victoria's second daughter, Alice, was dying of diphtheria. Princess Alice had spent the last weeks of her life in a petrified fugue, tending to her brood of children and her husband as they all lay desperately ill. Her youngest daughter, May, passed away from the disease that had steadily stalked the family. Thirty-five-year-old Alice followed her little girl to the grave when the diphtheria membrane cut off her breathing and choked her to death.

In the 1800s, even the privileged life of a princess was no protection against the blight of deadly infectious diseases such as diphtheria. Perhaps the most shocking aspect of her death was how truly universal it was. Princess Alice's experience was by no means unique. People died from diphtheria in tenements. They died in castles, in the sooty air of industrial London, and in the fresher air of the German countryside. They died as babies, as children, as adolescents, as young adults, as mature members of the community, and in old age.

But mostly they died as babies and children.

Before a vaccine was developed in the 1920s, diphtheria was one of the most feared of all childhood diseases. People called it "the strangling angel of children."[1] As one source notes, even as late as 1937, "diphtheria was second only to pneumonia among all causes of death in children," even in advanced industrialized countries such as England and Wales.[2] Treatments did little good. The only protection was quarantine once the first case appeared. Healthy members of the family would be sent away if possible, while sufferers took to their beds for weeks and courted death with every deep breath.

Diphtheria was but one of many serious childhood diseases that petrified mothers for centuries. The average life span was shorter for much of history for a simple reason: vaccine-preventable diseases that killed children early. Measles, mumps, influenza, pertussis, rubella, and other diseases are often far more deadly to babies and children than to adults. An adult might fight off illness and eventually walk away a little weaker and perhaps with less sharp eyesight and a few missing brain cells but still indisputably alive.

Babies often had no such luck even in places with good sanitation and effective nursing care. To use only a single endemic childhood disease as an example, whooping cough (pertussis) hits small children and tiny infants particularly hard. Most adults endure it, cough for a little while, and move on. Before the introduction of the whooping cough vaccine nearly two million Americans caught whooping cough in the 1920s.[3] An average of 7,300 hundred people died annually as a result. The majority of the dead were babies and children. Comparable figures during the 1980s (after the introduction of the vaccine) are thirty-five thousand cases and only fifty-six total deaths.[4]

Surviving childhood before vaccines most often meant battling dozens of diseases in a few short years. A baby's vulnerable immune system yielded easily to natural bacterial infections. The sheer number of diseases at the time meant babies coped with repeated encounters with potentially deadly diseases dozens of times a month. No societies or classes were spared. Even in an industrially advanced country such as England, "as late as 1899, more than 16 percent of all children did not survive to their first birthday."[5]

Ultimately in a very real sense, the history of the world is the history of parents losing babies again and again and again to vaccine-preventable diseases.

For much of recorded history, contraceptives were both ineffective and very hard to get. Becoming a woman meant getting married, and being married was synonymous with becoming a mother. Many societies did not allow a married woman to legally refuse her husband's sexual advances. As a result, to be married and fertile not only meant babies but lots of them. Many fertile women spent decades either pregnant, recovering from childbirth, or nursing. Queen Victoria, exemplifying the fate of women throughout history, had nine children.

Another important aspect of becoming a mother was to give birth to babies who did not survive childhood. Mothers went through life expecting to watch at least one and probably several of their babies cough furiously or develop a rash or high fever and then die before leaving the cradle. A baby might die for the same reasons they die today, such as a birth defect or obstructed bowel. But babies usually died from vaccine-preventable diseases.

The experience of bearing babies and losing them was so common that people coined a phrase to describe it: a real mother.

A real mother was someone who listened as her newborn began the characteristic whooping sound that marked a baby turning blue from whooping cough. A real mother was a woman who sat helplessly as her children broke out in spots from smallpox that could kill within a week. A real mother looked for signs of measles in her babies, praying that the disease would pass without inflaming their brains.

Caring for desperately ill babies and children was not a simple matter of soothing a feverish brow or gently rocking a fussy baby back to sleep. Watching over a baby with pertussis or a small child with measles required constant care and effort. Mothers expected to be on duty with sick family members twenty-four hours a day. Successfully steering a baby or child through a serious illness often left them no other choice. A baby dehydrated from throwing up for an hour required a mother who could provide him with access to fresh breast milk to help avoid convulsions. If the child was not expected to recover, mothers sat at the deathbed for hours, anxiously waiting for the final death rattle.

A brood of children struck with measles needed physical as well as mental comforts. Soiled beds needed clean linens to help prevent the spread of germs from patients to healthy family members. Recovering children needed nourishing foods that could be easily digested, such as broths. Quiet rooms where convalescents could rest peacefully and get sleep were essential to allow patients the rest necessary for a full recovery. In a world where hot water was scarce and people's lodgings often consisted of a single room, these conditions were very hard to meet for most people. Fabrics were expensive as well as extremely difficult to launder. Access to uncontaminated, high-quality ingredients to help patients get adequate nutrition was beyond the fiscal reach of a great many people, especially if an illness occurred during the winter months when fruits and vegetables were rarely available. Doctors charged expensive fees and often did little good.

The ever-present threat of vaccine-preventable diseases always held out the daunting prospect that mothers could find themselves facing months of constant care at a moment's notice. A disease such as smallpox created the need for skilled nursing for as long as several months. Mothers were expected to be available to care for seriously ill family members for as long as it took for them to get better. Getting a baby through a bout of influenza often meant many weeks at his side without knowing when he would shake off the illness or succumb to it. On a cold day, a weary mother might find herself constantly lighting fires in her child's room as she struggled to keep him warm. A hot summer night might make it harder to bring down a high fever.

Family members who recovered and no longer needed around-the-clock nursing often needed yet more months of supervision and assistance. An attack of measles could leave a child barely capable of getting out of bed for a prolonged period. Scrupulous supervision was required lest the child's weakened constitution make her vulnerable to illness yet again. Recovery from many vaccine-preventable diseases often took weeks if not months. A child who no longer had hundreds of scabbed pustules from smallpox all over her body still required weeks to regain her full health.

Even a single sick child in the house added almost immeasurably to a mother's workload. Before the industrial revolution, most women worked at home with their families. Her duties typically included sewing the family's clothing, tending to the family's animals, making staples such as butter and cheese, and cooking most meals. A baby with whooping cough or measles or diphtheria was a baby who required even more additional tasks the mother had to complete on a daily basis. Many women had help caring for sick children from older children or other family members. Others faced the Herculean prospect of watching over the entire family and attempting to complete their daily chores during the course of the illness. A farm that went untended was a farm that would not bring food or income the family needed to avoid starvation.

After the industrial revolution, caring for sick children became even harder for many women. While the countryside and farm at least brought fresh air and a network of reliable extended family members to help out in times of need, the pollution-filled skies of London, New York, and Paris offered no such safety nets. To pursue economic opportunity was often to pursue it in unfamiliar surroundings. Most people had even less access to clean water in the inner city. Crowded tenements allowed disease to spread quickly from one house to another. Mothers who faced the need to help feed their families would have to make the harsh choice of enlisting a younger member of the family to care for a sick child or work fewer hours and confront nutrition deficits and lost income.

The medicine of the time had almost nothing to offer to help. Indeed, treatments such as bleeding or noxious chemicals applied to the skin or taken internally often made disease worse. Mothers turned to other parents and members of the community for help as well. A grandmother might have a list of herbal remedies that could alleviate minor symptoms such as fever or headache. However, no remedies existed for more serious problems such as lungs filled with fluid from pneumonia or the convulsions that marked tetanus. Mothers could only watch, worry, pray, and spend hours watching a child's face for signs that a fever was breaking or listening for a cough that no longer shook their baby's entire body.

Perhaps worst of all, they could only wait for the next illness that would be sure to arrive at an unknown time. Reading a list of vaccine-preventable diseases before vaccines was like reading a list of common ancient curses. Many mothers could easily name most commonly known vaccine-preventable diseases as if reciting a list of the ten plagues during a Passover Seder: diphtheria, measles, mumps, smallpox, tetanus, and whooping cough. Each disease carried a particular list of horrors that mothers had to be prepared to confront.

Many children and babies would recover from a vaccine-preventable illness only to face a debilitating complication. Smallpox might attack the eyes, leaving the survivor blind. The disease could attack the joints, leaving people with painful arthritis. The disease could create a face full of pitted scars, and a woman with a pockmarked face was often shunted away from a chance at education and marriage. A bout of mumps could swell a little boy's testicles and cause unexpected infertility later in life. Measles can steal hearing. Meningitis from a bacterium such as Hib can bring about permanent mental impairment. Famed *Little House on the Prairie* author Laura Ingalls Wilder's husband contracted diphtheria and had a stroke that left him partially paralyzed for the rest of his life.[6] In the age before vaccines, millions were left with severe problems long after the actual disease was nothing but an unpleasant half-remembered childhood experience. Millions of people face similar potential complications today in areas where vaccines remain too expensive to easily obtain.

Some vaccine-preventable diseases offered one advantage for survivors. Once patients recovered, they would be immune for life. Other diseases, such as diphtheria, polio, and tetanus, offered no such benefits. A child could get sick, survive, and then get sick again with the exact same disease.

Many diseases of this period have faded into historical memory in most modern societies. Typhoid and cholera have been largely eliminated with safer and cleaner water supplies. Scarlet fever, the result of an advanced case of strep throat, is easily cured by modern antibiotics before the disease progresses that far. Many other feared illnesses are no longer seen in the developed world because of widespread usage of vaccines.

VACCINE-PREVENTABLE DISEASES

Chicken Pox

Chicken pox is a highly infectious illness caused by the varicella zoster virus. The primary symptom is an itchy rash that can quickly spread all over an infected person's body and lasts for about a week. Other typical symptoms include headache and fever. Infected individuals can get the rash anywhere, including the scalp, mouth, and even eyelids. If scratched, the pox can leave lifelong scars. Before the introduction of the vaccine in the United States, about ten thousand children were hospitalized annually because of the illness.[7] Approximately one hundred kids died each year.[8]

Chicken pox is a mildly unpleasant disease for most kids. They will get through it without problems. Unfortunately, the disease is far more dangerous for many vulnerable populations. Pregnant mothers who have not had a case of the disease in childhood and have not gotten the vaccine can get chicken pox and pass it on to their fetuses. Babies in the womb that are infected with chicken pox are at high risk for a disease known as congenital varicella syndrome (CVS). When the fetus is infected before twenty-eight weeks gestation, CVS can cause all kinds of serious birth defects in babies including brain damage, cataracts, and spinal cord abnormalities.

Adults who get chicken pox also face much higher risks of complications than children do, such as pneumonia and encephalitis. Chicken pox also poses a much greater risk of serious side effects for babies, children, and adults who are immunocompromised, such as HIV patients or transplant patients.

Infected individuals also face a much greater risk of a disease known as shingles. Shingles is a reactivation of the zoster virus in the body decades after the disease has passed. When the virus flares up, it can attack nerves, causing tremendous pain for many sufferers. The risk of a case of shingles can be greatly reduced by getting a shingles vaccine.

Diphtheria

Diphtheria is a highly infectious disease caused by bacteria. People can easily transmit the illness by coughing and sharing personal items such as drinking glasses and toys. Sufferers begin showing symptoms two to five days after an infection. Common symptoms include fever, sore throat, and chills. The most infected areas of the body are the neck and throat. When the neck is affected, a person may develop very swollen glands—a symptom known as bull neck. When the throat is affected, a thick covering can form over the back of the throat, making it very difficult to breathe.

A second form of the illness, known as cutaneous diphtheria, can also occur. Cutaneous, or skin, diphtheria is seen more often in tropical areas. This form can cause large, painful skin ulcers to break out across the legs or arms.

While many people experience disagreeable but not serious symptoms, the illness can cause life-threatening side effects. The diphtheria toxin may spread from a patient's throat to the rest of the organs including the heart and kidneys. During a bout of diphtheria, people may become temporarily paralyzed from nerve damage, unable to breathe without a respirator, suffering lifelong complications as a result.

Before the advent of vaccines, diphtheria was a familiar and extremely terrifying illness with a long and highly documented history. Greek physician Hippocrates provided an accurate clinical description of the disease as early as the fourth century B.C.[9] The Spanish dubbed it "el garatillo," or the strangler, while the Italians called diphtheria the gullet disease.[10]

Without modern treatment methods such as respirators and intravenous fluids, between one-third and one-half of all diphtheria patients could expect to die. Even today with access to state-of-the-art treatments, diphtheria still causes a roughly one in ten fatality rate.[11] Children and the elderly are particularly susceptible to the diphtheria toxin. While adults in the prime of life face a 5 percent death rate, estimated death rates for kids under five and older adults are as high as 20 percent.[12]

In the prevaccine era, diphtheria hit all socioeconomic classes. Frank and Lillian Gilbreth, the pioneering industrial engineers depicted in the beloved children's novel *Cheaper By the Dozen*, lost one of their children to a diphtheria epidemic. Outbreaks of the illness occurred quite frequently around the world. As late as the 1920s, Americans coped with over a hundred thousand cases each year and more than ten thousand deaths.[13] By the 1910s science could finally offer patients two treatments. Patients could be injected with an antitoxin to reduce some symptoms. Patients who did not respond well to the injection and then experienced further progression of the disease could also be helped with the insertion of tubes to help them breathe.

German scientist Emil von Behring won the first Nobel Prize in medicine for isolating the diphtheria toxin. By 1913, Behring had developed a vaccine for diphtheria. Once the vaccine came into widespread use, the number of cases began to fall. Cases in the United States are extremely rare today. Health officials typically see less than a hundred such cases each year.[14]

Diphtheria still remains a problem in the developing world. In the 1990s, more than three thousand people came down with the disease in Russia in the aftermath of governmental upheaval.[15] Today, the World Health Organization still expects to confront roughly four thousand cases each year worldwide.[16]

Hib

The near eradication of Hib disease from American shores is a modern-day medical triumph. Before the introduction and widespread use of a vaccine, Hib disease was a nightmare that both parents and pediatricians dreaded. Each year more than twenty thousand babies and children nationwide would get sick from Hib infection.[17] More than a thousand could be expected to die from it.[18] Hundreds more children under two would develop major complications that included reduced mental capacity, paralysis, deafness, and arthritis.[19]

Hib disease still remains a significant source of infant mortality in the developing world. More than three million babies and children get Hib disease each year in countries with low per capita income, resulting in hundreds of thousands of utterly needless deaths.[20] Efforts by public health officials are under way to fund widespread low-cost access to the vaccine in dozens of countries.

Hib is a very hazardous disease that can cause long-lasting side effects in children under five. It is caused by a contagious bacterium known as *Haemophilius influenzae*. First identified in 1892 by German bacteriologist Richard Pfeiffer, the bacterium has six forms that have been classified from a through f. The form of the bacteria that is the most dangerous to humans is known as Hib, or *Haemophilius influenzae* type b. Humans can easily spread the infection with a single cough or sneeze.

A baby or young child infected with Hib may develop horrible complications including meningitis, joint infections, pneumonia, and skin infections. Babies may also be at serious risk of epiglottitis. Epiglottitis is an infection of the cartilage at the back of the tongue. The infection can lead to swelling that can make it difficult for a baby to breathe. Infants with epiglottitis must be admitted to a hospital as soon as possible for treatment of the infection or else risk suffocation. In the era before the vaccine, mastering the effective treatment of epiglottitis was an essential skill for all pediatricians.

The most common complication of Hib remains meningitis. More than half of individuals infected with Hib will develop this highly dangerous swelling of the membranes covering the brain.[21] Meningitis is a medical emergency. Even with treatment, death will still occur in one out of every twenty patients.[22] Meningitis survivors face frightening aftereffects. Nearly one in four will suffer from long-term brain damage.[23] A particularly severe case of Hib disease can lead to death in less than a single day.

Many infants have some form of initial protection against Hib disease from their mothers. Breastfeeding has been shown to confer some immunity to Hib but still leaves infants highly vulnerable to infection in the event of an outbreak.[24] Since Hib disease typically peaks between six months and two years, babies left unprotected either due to a lack of vaccines or a lack of access to vaccines can get sick if they encounter the bacteria outside the womb. Worse still, bouts of Hib can recur, as getting the disease in infancy does not provide immunity against a recurrence in babies under two.[25]

Fortunately, the vaccine is very effective. About 95 percent of babies who are given the recommended three doses will develop antibodies to provide protection against infection during this crucial period and for many years afterward.[26]

HPV

The initials HPV stand for human papillomavirus. HPV is one of a family of extremely common infections. These viruses can lead to minor health issues such as plantar warts as well as more serious problems, including genital warts and invasive reproductive cancers. Nearly two hundred forms of the virus are known to exist. Each type is referred to by a number. Roughly thirty to forty types of HPV are believed to be transmitted by sexual contact. As a result, half of all sexually active men and women can expect to get at least one form of HPV in their lifetimes.[27]

HPV infection is known to increase the risk of getting cervical cancer, vaginal cancer, penile cancer, anal cancer, and cancers of the neck, head, and throat. An HPV infection can also increase one's risk of genital warts.

Researchers seek to reduce the spread of HPV and to help prevent infection by the most virulent types of the virus. In 2006, the FDA approved a vaccine known as Gardasil. The Gardasil vaccine protects against four types of HPV: types 6, 11, 16, and 18. The first two carry a high risk of causing genital warts. The latter two types can vastly increase a woman's chances of developing cervical cancer. The use of the vaccine should reduce a woman's odds of developing cervical cancer by more than two-thirds.[28] However, the vaccine does not protect against all known forms of HPV.

Hepatitis B

Hepatitis B is one of five viruses that can cause inflammation of the liver. Long-term inflammation may have serious side effects including the eventual need for a liver transplant. Cases of hepatitis have been documented for centuries. Historical outbreaks were more common during times of crisis such as war and famine. In modern times, hepatitis B infection has become extremely widespread. According to the Hepatitis B Foundation, "Hepatitis B is 100 times more infectious than the AIDS virus."[29] More than two billion people worldwide are infected with the disease.[30] Hundreds of people across the globe acquire the infection each day. Even in the United States, health officials estimate that more than twelve million people, or roughly one in twenty Americans, are infected with hepatitis B.[31] Many of them do not know they are infected.

Hepatitis B is traditionally divided into acute and chronic infections. Acute infections often induce symptoms such as vomiting and jaundice but eventually pass from the body without usually causing any lasting physical damage. Additional symptoms include loss of appetite, itchy skin, and constant low-grade fever. Chronic hepatitis B infections have the same symptoms but are far more likely to cause lasting problems including cirrhosis and liver cancer. One of the most troubling aspects of hepatitis B infection is that some individuals may be infected without any symptoms at all. As a result, it is easily possible for you and your child to be exposed to someone with hepatitis B and not even be aware of it.

Hepatitis B poses several unique problems for infants. The primary problem is that most infants cannot pass the infection from their bodies. While the vast majority of adults can recover without progressing to a chronic infection, only 30 to 50 percent of children under five will be able to pass the virus from their systems.[32] The odds are even worse for infected newborns. About 90 percent of all infected newborns will not be able to rid themselves of the virus once infected.[33]

A baby infected with hepatitis B usually does not have any initial symptoms. Many, however, will eventually experience serious problems from the infection that vastly increase their chances of both liver failure and liver cancer.

Fortunately, hepatitis B is difficult to spread. Most individuals acquire cases of hepatitis B from sexual contact and sharing items with an infected person. A baby may become infected during birth if his mother has been infected. However, not all methods of infection are understood. As many as 30 percent of all infected individuals have no known risk factors.[34] Therefore, people can harbor the infection and pass it on to others without showing symptoms or knowing they are infected.

A vaccine for the hepatitis B virus was developed in the early 1980s. Pediatricians recommend that all babies get the vaccine, as not all risk factors for transmission are understood. The vaccine is given in three doses. The first dose is administered within twelve hours of birth. Three doses provide decades of immunity to hepatitis B for most infants. Millions of doses of the vaccine have been given to children and adults around the world since then. Serious side effects seen from the vaccine have been quite rare.

Influenza

Influenza, or the flu, is a very infectious disease that recurs seasonally. The flu shows up during the winter months and then abates as warmer weather approaches. Pandemics of influenza have spread through communities throughout the world for hundreds of years. Europeans battled epidemics of influenza repeatedly during the seventeenth and eighteenth centuries. In 1918, a famous and utterly terrifying two-year outbreak of the flu swept across the world. From Antarctica to the peaceful Pacific islands, no corner of the planet was exempt from the disease. Scientists and historians estimate that at least twenty million and as many as one hundred million people probably died during this short period.[35]

The flu remains a modern-day threat as well. Hundreds of thousands of people continue to come down with influenza each year. The Centers for Disease Control and Prevention estimates that two hundred thousand Americans will need hospitalization as a result of the flu, with as many as forty-nine thousand annual deaths.[36]

Influenza can be spread quickly by casual contact with another person such as sharing tissues or sneezing on someone. Typical flu symptoms include high fever, chills, body aches, headache, and nasal congestion. A case of the illness can progress to more serious complications including extreme fatigue, pneumonia, abdominal pain, and shortness of breath.

Children under five are more vulnerable to influenza than adults. They catch it more easily and get sicker from it than adults do. Babies and children under five are also more likely to suffer more severe consequences from the flu if they get the disease. Small children with weakened immune systems as a result of other conditions such as HIV or asthma face increased risks of complications if infected.

Children are also susceptible to the effects of the flu when still in the womb. Miscarriages and premature labor are more common in women who have been infected. A study has shown higher rates of schizophrenia in the children of mothers who have the flu when pregnant.[37]

In the 1940s, American scientists developed a vaccine for the flu. Since then doctors have recommended the vaccine for babies over six months. Making the flu vaccine is a complex yearly process. Before the beginning of flu season, world health officials gather to assess information about expected strains of the virus. Once a consensus has been reached, vaccine production begins. The vaccine is usually ready for use by early fall.

Use of the vaccine helps protect people against getting the illness and also reduces the severity of symptoms in people if they do catch it. People can get the flu vaccine via an injection of a killed virus or from a nasal spray. The nasal spray contains a very weakened form of the virus. The nasal spray method is useful for children older than two years, letting them avoid the sting of a shot. Pregnant women are particularly vulnerable to the flu. A flu shot can help reduce her chances of getting the flu and can also protect her unborn child. A study in the October 4, 2011, edition of *Archives of Pediatrics*

& Adolescent Medicine found that mothers who had a flu shot greatly reduced the risk that their babies would develop the flu in the first six months of life.[38] As babies cannot get vaccinated for the flu during this period, this vaccine can offer protection for both mother and baby.

Measles

Measles is one of the world's most contagious infections. Caused by a virus known as a paramyxovirus, the disease has threatened humanity for thousands of years. Measles has a long and ugly history that is still, alas, being played out today.

Historically, measles epidemics would periodically sweep through many communities every two to five years. Inhabitants of small villages and large cities would recover from the disease only to get hit with it again. While largely initially confined to the European continent, measles was spread around the world when Europeans began to travel across the Atlantic. Explorers and colonists brought the illness to the New World, often without knowing it. Natives had no natural immunity. Thousands of indigenous people died in all corners of both North and South America. Medical investigators estimate that more than two hundred million people have died from measles infection in the last two centuries.[39]

Before a vaccine was developed in the 1960s, nearly every single person could expect to get measles during her lifetime. If your neighbor, friend, mother, father, sister, or classmates had measles, the enormous odds were that you would get it as well—and get it quite soon. This was not a good thing for most people and their children. Author Roald Dahl, writer of such children's classics as *Charlie and the Chocolate Factory*, watched with deepest sorrow as his eldest daughter died shortly after coming down what was thought to be a mild case. The heir to the French throne and his wife caught measles in the 1700s and died a short while later.

Individuals who catch measles still often have huge problems as a result. Today, even otherwise relatively healthy people in developed countries face a nearly one in three risk of complications if they get measles.[40] Common measles symptoms include high fever, an itchy rash that can spread all over the body, conjunctivitis (pinkeye), and sore throat. People infected with measles are also at high risk from more severe complications including pneumonia, middle ear infections that may lead to hearing loss, and a measles-induced inflammation of brain tissue known as measles encephalitis.

Young babies often have temporary immunity as mothers pass their antibodies to the disease to their newborns. Unfortunately, older babies and children under five are particularly susceptible to the illness and any side effects.[41] Hospitalization is frequently recommended to make sure individuals get enough fluid and rest. The only known treatment for measles infection is an increased dose of vitamin A. Individuals infected with measles who do not ultimately rid themselves of the infection are further at risk of developing SSPE, or subacute sclerosing panencephalitis. SSPE is a fatal disease caused by ongoing measles infection of the brain.

The development and widespread use of the vaccine have had enormous effects on the number of measles cases across the globe. Many developed nations have seen the number of measles cases drop drastically. Before the vaccine, over half a million people caught measles each year in the United States alone. Since then most American children no longer break out in itchy spots as a rite of passage. Parents no longer hover near a child's sickbed worrying about measles encephalitis and potential brain damage. Worldwide cases of measles have fallen to below two hundred thousand annually as efforts to introduce the vaccine have become more widespread.[42] With continued vaccination, measles may even be eradicated from the planet one day in the same way that smallpox has been.

Unfortunately, a campaign of misinformation about the vaccine has led parents to shy away from it. As a result, the number of measles cases continues to rise in many nations. Thousands of children have come down with measles in Europe. In the United States, measles outbreaks have been reported in dozens of communities that were previously free of the disease. While deaths have been quite rare in both regions, measles infection typically requires hospitalization for more than 40 percent of all infected individuals.[43] In light of this campaign of misinformation, public health officials have stepped up efforts to convince parents to continue to vaccinate their children.

Mumps

Mumps is a very contagious infectious disease caused by a virus. Cases of mumps have been documented in the historical literature for centuries. The name of the illness is said to derive from an older word for lumps. Mumps may have been named because of the inflammation of the parotid salivary glands that is the hallmark of the disease. These glands are located adjacent to the jawbone. As a result of mumps infection, the glands can swell up quite painfully, making it difficult for patients to swallow, chew, and even talk.

Adults can come down with mumps, but the disease is primarily found in children over a year and in younger adolescents. Mumps can spread from person to person by coughing, sneezing, and sharing a cup or spoon with an infected person. The illness can cause many potentially dangerous symptoms in children including fever, headache, sore throat, earache, and aching joints.

Adolescent males who catch it face the potential risk of a particular complication known as mumps orchitis, in which the testicles can become agonizingly swollen. This condition can linger for days and occasionally, although rarely, results in sterility. Adolescent girls face a similar possibility that their ovaries may also swell up as a result of mumps infection.

Mumps can also cause miscarriage, meningitis, pancreatitis, and hearing loss in certain individuals. Mumps has no specific treatment or cure. Treatment consists of giving pain relievers and watching the patient closely to see if more serious complications develop as the disease runs its course.

A vaccine for mumps was developed in the late 1960s. With widespread use of the vaccine, cases of mumps in the United States have fallen from over two hundred thousand each year to less than five hundred cases annually.[44] The disease is more widespread in developing countries where access to the mumps vaccine is limited. Officials had aimed to eliminate the disease from the United States by 2010. Unfortunately, in recent years, vaccine refusal and the need for a more effective vaccine as well as perhaps a booster shot has helped push the number of cases up. In 2006, nearly seven thousand Americans came down with a case of the mumps.[45]

Pertussis (Whooping Cough)

Pertussis is a very infectious illness caused by a dangerous bacterial infection. Pertussis is also known as whooping cough because the disease causes patients to cough so severely that the sound they make sounds like a "whoop" noise to observers. Patients can cough so violently they can pass out or break a bone. While many adults can get through a bout of whooping cough as they would an ordinary cold, babies and children can easily get much sicker from infection.

Symptoms of pertussis infection include runny nose, fever, and a deep cough. The painful cough characteristic of the disease can continue to show up and cause suffering for weeks on end. As a result the ancient Chinese dubbed pertussis the one-hundred-day cough. While coughing is rare in babies under six months, older babies and children can cough so forcefully they can turn blue during the cough or even break a rib.

The pertussis incubation period may be as long as three weeks from infection to the start of active symptoms. Once infected, the paroxysmal stage can last over two months. This is when people with the illness can cough hard enough to gasp for air or vomit. Patients typically burst into a series of prolonged coughs that can strain their lungs and make it almost impossible to breathe.

After the paroxysmal stage, the patient enters the convalescent stage, when the symptoms begin to subside. However, patients can still experience severe spells of coughing. A new cold or minor infection during this stage can trigger renewed severe coughing bouts. The convalescent stage can last for months.

Complications from pertussis may be serious and long lasting. Sufferers are prone to pneumonia, rib fractures, ear infections, and dehydration during the course of the disease.

If the disease is diagnosed within the first two weeks of infection, symptoms can be greatly reduced with the use of antibiotics. However, early symptoms of pertussis can be hard to distinguish from a simple cough or cold. People with milder symptoms can spread whooping cough unknowingly. Babies under six months with pertussis are usually hospitalized so they can be watched closely. Treatment consists of palliative measures such as the administration of antibiotics, steroids, IV fluids, and oxygen. A baby may be placed on a ventilator if the disease continues to worsen. Children under two are most at risk of complications from pertussis.

Infection is thought to provide immunity from further disease for up to seven years. Adults and children can get ill more than once.

Pertussis typically breaks out in three- to five-year cycles. During a peak year, health officials expect to see thousands of cases. Vaccination efforts can help greatly reduce these numbers. Babies are given five doses of the whooping cough vaccine starting at two months. Even a single dose can provide crucial protection against the disease. Babies who have been partially vaccinated will more than likely be at least somewhat protected against pertussis and have lessened symptoms if they later catch the illness.

Children and adolescents should be given booster shots because the vaccine can wear off in less than ten years. Some doctors also recommend an additional shot for adults, especially if they are involved in childcare.

Until the introduction of the vaccine, whooping cough was a serious public health threat. As late as the 1940s, health authorities believe there were approximately 150,000 cases annually and thousands of deaths.[46] Most of the dead were infants under six months. Since that time, the number of pertussis cases has abated, largely due to the vaccine. In fact, for a period of time, most people never gave whooping cough a second thought. Many people grew up without even knowing the name of the disease. In recent years, however, a campaign of misinformation regarding the vaccine has caused a reduction in vaccination rates, primarily because of unfounded fears. This has led to a resurgence of the disease in many nations including the United States. The number of cases has more than doubled in some states. In California in 2010, more than nine thousand cases of whooping cough were reported. Ten infants died. The return of this deadly disease makes vaccination more imperative than ever.

Polio

Polio is a viral infection that can cause paralysis and death. Worldwide polio outbreaks have been documented since the 1840s. In the first five decades of the 1900s, periodic epidemics would sweep across the United States. In 1952, at the height of the pandemic, there were more than fifty thousand cases nationwide and three thousand deaths.[47] While polio strikes people of any age, children are particularly prone to infection. Prior to the development of the polio vaccine, many parents spent summers worrying that their children would come home one day with a stiff neck or a fever and spend the rest of their lives in a wheelchair or iron lung. Doctors could do little to tell parents how to avoid infection. Treatment even today consists of supportive measures such as the use of ventilators to help patients breathe and physical therapy afterward to help patients regain as much range of motion as possible in paralyzed limbs.

Perhaps the most famous American polio victim is Franklin Roosevelt. Our only four-term president came down with the illness in his twenties. Despite years of trying out various therapies, Roosevelt never walked unaided even after he no longer had any other symptoms.

Poliovirus can cause three different types of infection: subclinical, paralytic, and nonparalytic. While most people are infected without showing symptoms (subclinical infection), approximately one in twenty patients will show some signs of illness. Those signs can range from fever and sore throat to meningitis-like symptoms or paralysis that often requires hospitalization to treat. Paralytic polio is the most serious form of the disease. About two in a hundred people who get infected from poliovirus experience muscle paralysis and the real possibility of dying without swift medical treatment.[48] Survivors of paralytic polio often deal with severe pain from aching and immobilized muscles. A minority of patients spent their lives living in iron lungs because the illness left them unable to breathe on their own ever again.

An effective vaccine was developed in the 1950s. Since that time, the number of cases of polio has fallen rapidly. Polio has largely been eradicated from the Western hemisphere. Massive vaccination efforts are reducing the incidence of the disease in the rest of the world as well.

Rotavirus

Rotavirus is an extremely common infection that strikes young children. Nearly all children will have at least one bout of the illness before they are three. While most cases of rotavirus are minor, the disease can progress to more serious side effects in many children.

Named for the shape of the virus (*rota* is Latin for wheel), rotavirus can be found all over the world. The virus attacks the digestive system and causes symptoms such as fever and abdominal pain. Infants generally get through it with nothing more than a few days of fussiness. However, more severe cases can result in watery diarrhea that leads to dangerous side effects from dehydration. Rotavirus causes over half a million deaths in children under five each year in the developing world.

A vaccine was introduced in the United States in 2006. Before the introduction of the vaccine, one in seven children went to a doctor each year in the United States as a result of the virus, and one in fifty were hospitalized.[49] A few dozen of these children died of rotavirus infection. The vaccine has helped push down these numbers and reduce mortality rates in the countries where the vaccine is available. In countries where it is not, officials estimate that over five hundred thousand children die each year as a result.[50]

Rubella

Rubella is a viral infection. Also known as German measles to distinguish it from traditional measles, rubella is usually a mild illness that often passes unnoticed by most people. The most common rubella symptom is a rash that begins on the face and spreads across the rest of the upper body. The rash typically fades after three days. People can also experience low-grade fever, headaches, and swollen glands.

The illness is rare in infants and older adults. While most adults and children who get rubella suffer no ill effects, the disease can have devastating side effects for pregnant women and the fetuses they carry.

When rubella infects a pregnant woman in the first trimester or second trimester, congenital rubella syndrome (CRS) can result. CRS can cause all kinds of serious side effects in fetuses. Many women miscarry if they come into contact with the virus. The babies that survive are often born with severe side effects including deafness, blindness, and mental retardation.

Before the development of the vaccine, outbreaks of CRS were common. In the 1960s, more than twelve million cases of CRS were documented.[51] More than twenty thousand infants developed CRS.[52] Thousands of children were born deaf, blind, or mentally retarded as a result of the infection. In 1943, Academy Award-nominated actress Gene Tierney gave birth to a daughter with multiple birth defects as a result of CRS. Her daughter was infected when an ardent fan slipped out of quarantine for German measles and hugged the pregnant actress.

Widespread implementation of the vaccine has led to the elimination of rubella from many countries. Continued use of the rubella vaccine should help push down the number of cases even further.

Smallpox

Smallpox was once possibly the world's most feared disease. The disease is both extremely contagious and highly debilitating. In its most common form, smallpox kills nearly one in three who catch it. Survivors often emerged from weeks of sickness blind, arthritic, or deformed from severe scarring across much of their skin.

Today the illness exists only in laboratories and historical memory. The vaccine is used only for some members of the military and not for the general population.

Tetanus

Tetanus is an infectious disease that causes extremely painful muscle spasms. Left untreated, tetanus has a nearly 25 percent mortality rate.[52] The disease is caused by the *Clostridium tetani* bacteria. People can contract tetanus if spores containing the bacterium enter the body from a puncture wound. Tetanus is one of the few vaccine-preventable diseases that is infectious but not contagious.

Tetanus is also known as lockjaw because the illness causes facial muscle spasms that are particularly noticeable in a person's jaw. The illness can be divided into four types: generalized tetanus, neonatal tetanus, local tetanus, and cephalic tetanus. The generalized form is the most common version. Neonatal tetanus strikes newborns and young babies. It most often results when expectant mothers deliver in unsanitary conditions where tetanus spores are present. Fatality rates for neonatal tetanus are extremely high.

Thanks to widespread vaccination, fewer than fifty Americans get tetanus each year.[53] Immunization also allows antibodies to the disease to be passed along from a mother to her baby. In places where the vaccine remains difficult to get, thousands of babies die each year from the neonatal form of the disease.

· 6 ·

The Worst-Case Scenario:
True Adverse Reactions

$\mathcal{I}$f you read any anti-vaccine literature, you could easily come away with one conclusion: a vaccine reaction is the worst possible thing that could ever happen to a baby. Worse, a vaccine reaction has the strong possibility of stripping your child's hearing or eyesight or personality or pushing your child into the well of autism. Much of this literature implies that dangerous vaccine reactions are incredibly common and pose a serious threat any time your child gets a shot. The literature claims there are hordes of vaccine-injured children the government and vaccine makers have ignored and left uncompensated.

The literature is wrong.

Let's be honest here. Vaccine reactions are not enjoyable for anyone, especially an already worried parent. Listening to your baby cry for an hour after he gets his measles, mumps, and rubella (MMR) shot may make you want to never let him go near any big, bad needles ever again. If you watch your child's leg develop a small lump a week after her second DTaP vaccine, you might swear off pediatric visits until your baby is old enough to head to college. While soothing a baby on an examining table, all parents know what's coming next. Even if you understand intellectually that vaccines are good and necessary, it's hard not to be just a bit unnerved at the sight of actual sharp pointy things about to enter your small baby's deliciously chubby thighs.

Vaccines are scary for many people for a simple reason: they can cause bad side effects. No one denies this fact. High fevers or fussiness or even a few dirty looks afterward as a result of receiving a vaccine are all considered vaccine reactions. A thorough understanding of the true odds of a reaction can help greatly reduce your fears and make the average pediatric visit less likely to induce panic attacks.

Reactions tend to be shrouded in mystery just a bit. One side claims that vaccine reactions are incredibly common and always very dangerous. The first part is true. Vaccine reactions are actually comparatively common. Some vaccines on the market have as high as a 50 percent chance of causing a minor physical problem afterward.

What the anti-vaccine literature won't tell you is that although vaccine reactions are very common, they're almost always harmless. A slight fever is no one's idea of fun, but it's not going to hurt your child a tenth as much as a case of Hib disease or the whole-body rash that many people get from the measles. The really bad reactions, the kind where your baby goes into convulsions and you rush to dial 911 five seconds later, are incredibly rare. So rare that decades of closely watched stats can barely find any such problems. Make no mistake: A few dozen health officials are looking for problems with vaccines every day of the year.

Doctors and scientists want to identify any potential problems with a specific shot or with the vaccine schedule. They don't want babies getting sick as a result of a vaccine. Every vaccine on the market has two aims: (1) protect the public from infectious diseases, and (2) reduce any potential side effects for everyone who gets it. The safest possible vaccine means a vaccine that works and does not cause physical problems, even for those at potentially high risk of a bad vaccine reaction.

SO WHAT IS A VACCINE REACTION?

A vaccine reaction is any unwanted side effect as a result of a vaccine. The purpose of a vaccine is to stimulate the immune system. When the immune system is stimulated to act, unexpected and unintended effects may occur. Scientists simply do not know exactly why some particular individuals are more likely to get a vaccine reaction than others. Some of the risk factors that may predispose an individual to a vaccine reaction include a prior individual or family history of vaccine reactions, a suppressed immune system, and allergies to certain vaccine ingredients. But not all reactions can be predicted. Someone with a family history of bad vaccine reactions may be just fine when given the recommended series of shots. Others without a family history may have a stronger reaction such as a high fever or a swollen arm.

In fact, it is possible for children to have a completely unexpected reaction to any medication, even a medication the child has received before. As a young child, Allison developed a condition known as Stevens-Johnson syndrome, which is a severe allergic reaction. It was probably triggered by the use of sulfa drugs. She completely lost her top layer of skin, spent days in the hospital with no treatment available other than supportive care, and spent weeks recovering. Luckily, there are usually only about three hundred cases of this condition diagnosed in the United States every year. The point is, reactions to vaccines are not unusual in comparison to reactions to other, more common medications that children receive all the time.

Health officials do know that someone at risk from a vaccine reaction is equally at risk should they get a vaccine-preventable illness. A killed form of a virus is hardly likely to provoke a less severe reaction than an actual full-blown case of the disease.

Side effects from vaccination can include fevers, chills, or soreness at the site of the injection. A baby might be fussier after a vaccine, or she might eat less or sleep more in the hours after she's been vaccinated. Toddlers can get clingier or eat and drink less after a series of shots. Some side effects can be immediate, such as fainting right after getting a vaccine. A vaccine reaction may also happen after a period of time such as few hours or even, rarely, a few days after the injection.

Health officials divide vaccine reactions into three categories: mild, moderate, and severe. **Mild side effects** are considered reactions that can be easily treated and that go away in a short period of time, such as a fever or swelling where the shot was given. Parents may not even notice reactions such as a slightly elevated temperature. **Moderate side effects** include prolonged crying fits, hives, and joint pains. Moderate side effects can usually be treated with low-level measures such as pain relievers. They can interfere with a person's normal activities but do not typically require medical attention and go away after a period of time. **Severe side effects** include pneumonia and seizures. Such side effects need immediate medical attention and can have detrimental long-term consequences.

Mild vaccine reactions are quite common. Moderate side effects are less so. Severe side effects happen, but they are extremely atypical. Any vaccine has the potential to cause a reaction in any given person. However, most reactions are minor and far less risky to any individual than the diseases the vaccines prevent. In short, your child can get a vaccine reaction. A mild vaccine reaction is easily treatable with a few physician-approved pain relievers. A mild vaccine reaction typically means no effects long term. Even if your child has a minor reaction such as bout of fussiness, that does not mean your child should not receive any additional vaccines or even multiple shots of the same vaccine spread out over time. Pediatricians still advise parents to complete the series of shots because the risks of vaccine-preventable diseases outweigh the risks of vaccine reactions.

The standard American vaccine schedule calls for shots to be given at various intervals. In early infancy, babies are given shots every two months.

Some parents believe they can reduce the possibility their baby will get a vaccine reaction by spreading out this schedule over a longer period of time. The problem with this argument is twofold.

First, some vaccines are given at an earlier age because young babies are more vulnerable to certain diseases. Whooping cough, for example, can often be shrugged off as a mere unpleasant cough in a ten-year-old. A ten-week-old baby with whooping cough is a medical emergency. Delaying vaccines merely increases the possibility that a baby will get the disease when he is most vulnerable. Second, delaying a vaccine does not reduce the possibility that a baby will react to it.[1] Your child will always have the same odds of reacting to a shot whether you give that shot at two months old or after the child's first birthday.

THE RISKS OF NONVACCINATION

Another important idea when examining vaccine reactions is the idea of risk. A risk is the possibility that something bad will happen. *Every single thing you do in life carries risks.* You cannot go through life without confronting risks.

From the moment you wake up to the moment you go to bed, your entire life in a sense is a series of risky events. This is simply an unavoidable fact of everyday life. As you get out of bed, you could fall and sprain your ankle or break your wrist if you roll out of bed too quickly. Take a shower and you could pull the lever too far in one direction and scald yourself. Even preparing a typical uncomplicated breakfast involves a series of hazards. The orange juice could have been left out too long on the counter and cause you an upset stomach (or even worse) if you drink it. You can burn your fingers if you reach into the toaster before the machine shuts off. Cut into rock-hard butter and you could slice into your thumb on the way down.

The risks hardly end when you step outside each day. Officials at the Harvard Center for Risk Analysis estimate the risk of getting into a car accident at one in 6,700 each year.[2]

None of these potential risks stop us from getting out of bed, taking showers, drinking orange juice, or buttering toast. Most people certainly don't think twice about driving their cars to work. They certainly don't think very much about the possibility of a car accident on the way to the pediatrician's office. Yet such risks, as uncommon as they may be, exist and always will.

The same kind of math should be applied to vaccines. Each vaccine-preventable disease and vaccine for that disease have several kinds of risks.

These include the odds of getting the actual illness and the risks of not vaccinating, as well as the risks of side effects from the vaccine.

The decision to forgo vaccines altogether, delay specific vaccines, or skip some shots and not others is also a form of risk taking. An outbreak of a vaccine-preventable illness may develop in your community without your knowing about it. Many vaccine-preventable illnesses are highly contagious. Even if the outbreak is publicized, health officials may not have enough vaccines immediately on hand to give to everyone. Vaccine shortages happen quite often. After your baby or child gets the vaccine, immunity can take time to develop leaving her still vulnerable to the illness.

Ultimately no matter what choice you make on vaccines, you are making a choice. You are still taking a risk whether you vaccinate or not.

The recommended vaccine schedule in most countries consists of thirty shots designed to protect babies and young children against fifteen diseases. Some babies may get more shots or fewer because of risk factors such as a parent's medical condition or the baby's prematurity. Some immunizations, such as the chicken pox, are less widely used in certain countries. But in general, most children will get vaccines designed to protect them against chicken pox, diphtheria, two forms of hepatitis, Hib, influenza, measles, meningitis, mumps, polio, pneumonia, rotavirus, rubella, tetanus, and whooping cough.

Some vaccines, such as the Hib, are designed to protect children against one disease with a single shot. Others, such as the MMR, contain multiple vaccines designed to protect children against several ailments with a single shot. Babies and children are usually given several shots in a row during a well-baby visit.

The odds of a child getting a vaccine-preventable disease depend on many differing factors. An unvaccinated mom who has hepatitis B carries a risk as high as 90 percent of transmitting the virus to her baby, depending on the particular form of the virus she carries.[3] In the middle of a whooping cough outbreak, just taking a baby to the local supermarket carries risks. Doing so can make it easier for the baby to come down with pertussis by exposing the infant to strangers who may carry the disease in milder form. Other risk factors that influence the possibility of getting a vaccine-preventable disease include one's geographic location, the year, a mother's prior vaccines or prior encounters with illness, and the number of people in the community who vaccinate their own children.

Some vaccine-preventable diseases are more common than others. Polio is very rare in the Western hemisphere, but cases have cropped up in Africa and Asia. Measles outbreaks have plagued Europe and India in recent decades. Vaccine-preventable diseases also go through cycles. Whooping cough cases spike roughly every five years.

In general, one must look at each disease individually and examine the odds of getting a severe vaccine reaction versus getting the disease.

Chicken pox is a widespread childhood disease that is still very much in circulation. Prior to the introduction of the vaccine in the 1990s, there were over three million cases of varicella each year.[4] The use of the vaccine has helped drive these numbers down drastically, but thousands of cases of chicken pox are still reported each year. An unvaccinated child can easily pick up the illness and come down with the disease. By contrast, the odds of having a severe reaction to the vaccine have been deemed "very low" by the CDC.[5]

Diphtheria was once an extremely common disease. The Alaskan Iditarod sled dog race from Anchorage to Nome was originally organized to combat a diphtheria epidemic in 1925. Diphtheria is an extremely rare disease today, with fewer than four thousand cases reported annually.[6] However, diphtheria is an illness with extremely high mortality rates and few methods of treatment. The vaccine for diphtheria is generally given as part of the DTaP vaccine, which is designed to also protect against tetanus and pertussis. The risk of an allergic reaction to this vaccine is estimated at less than one out of a million doses.[7]

Hepatitis A and B are two of the most common forms of hepatitis. Vaccines are given for each one. Hepatitis A is usually a mild form of hepatitis and does not lead to chronic disease. While the use of vaccines has driven down the number of new cases, health officials still estimate that more than twenty thousand people will be infected with this form of hepatitis annually. While the disease is almost never fatal, it can cause weeks of unpleasant symptoms including nausea, fever, diarrhea, and jaundice.[8] It is possible to have the disease without displaying any symptoms of infection. So the odds of getting the disease are quite high.

Hepatitis B is one of the most serious forms of hepatitis. Babies under five who get the disease will usually see it develop into the most serious kind that may require a liver transplant to cure. Before the vaccine, about thirty-three thousand babies each year were infected with the disease.[9] Even today, millions of people in the developing world carry the hepatitis B virus. Each vaccine carries minimal risk of a vaccine reaction. According to the CDC, "more than 100 million people have received Hepatitis B vaccine in the United States and no serious side effects have been reported."[10]

Hib is a disease that is significantly more dangerous to babies and children than to adults. Hib disease primarily causes meningitis but can cause other symptoms including pneumonia and agonizing throat infections. While Hib rates have fallen because of the introduction of the vaccine in 1987, Hib still lurks in the general population. Worldwide cases of Hib number in the millions, with hundreds of thousands of deaths each year. By contrast, the vaccine poses a very small risk of mild problems and an extremely low risk of serious side effects.

Influenza is a respiratory infection caused by the influenza virus. It is a seasonal infection that peaks during the winter. Each year more than a hundred thousand Americans will come down with the flu. Children under two are particularly at risk both from the illness and from potential complications should they catch it. An annual vaccine can greatly reduce a baby's risk of getting the disease and reduce symptoms if they occur. The risks of a bad reaction are extremely low. As the CDC reports, "Millions of doses of LAIV have been distributed since it was licensed, and the vaccine has not been associated with any serious problems."[11]

Measles is an ancient and extremely contagious disease. A bout of measles can cause reduced hearing, blindness, and encephalitis. The measles vaccine is given as part of the MMR vaccine. Without vaccination, nearly everyone who comes into contact with the disease will catch it. Measles cases were on the wane, but unjustified fears about the vaccine have driven cases upward. In the first three months of 2010 alone, French health officials were forced to cope with nearly five thousand cases of measles.[12] By the end of 2011, the number of cases of measles in France had more than tripled to over 15,000. Dozens of flights ferry people each day between most major American and French cities. A single infected individual from abroad can easily put babies at risk. In New Jersey, officials were forced to shut down a popular local restaurant for several days after two people from France showed up to a party and came down with measles a short while later. On the other hand, the risk of a severe vaccine reaction is less than one in a million.[13]

Meningitis is an inflammation of the membranes that cover the brain and spinal cord. Meningitis can be divided into bacterial meningitis and viral meningitis. A bout of meningitis is considered a medical emergency that must be treated as soon as possible. Without treatment, bacterial meningitis is nearly always fatal. Even with antibiotic treatment, bacterial meningitis has a mortality rate of greater than 10 percent.[14] Roughly four thousand cases are reported annually.[15] Two doses of the meningococcal vaccine (MCV4) are given during adolescence and offer high protection rates with very little risk.

Mumps is a highly contagious viral infection. A mumps infection can cause miscarriages, male infertility, hearing loss, and meningitis. As a result of the vaccine, mumps infections are extremely uncommon. However, outbreaks still happen periodically. In 2009, more than 1,500 cases were reported in the New York City area when a young boy caught the disease while visiting the United Kingdom.[16] The mumps vaccine is given with the vaccine for measles and rubella. The odds of a severe reaction to the vaccine are thought to be less than one in a million.[17]

Polio was once the scourge of American parents. Thousands of children were paralyzed by polio infection during the first five decades of the last century. Since the introduction of the vaccine the disease has nearly disappeared from the world. Pockets of infection still exist in some African and Asian nations, but officials are working to improve worldwide vaccination rates. The odds of contracting polio are nearly nil. Polio vaccination is divided into two types: the oral polio vaccine (OPV) and the inactivated polio vaccine (IPV). The OPV is slightly more effective at preventing polio than the IPV. However, the OPV carries a very small risk of causing paralysis because it is a live virus. Officials estimate paralysis risk from the use of the oral vaccine by itself at one out of every 750,000 doses.[18] Health officials have been using both vaccines. Two doses of the inactivated polio vaccine are administered followed by two doses of the oral polio vaccine later. The use of the IPV prevents the potential risk of paralysis from the OPV.[19]

Pneumonia is a very dangerous infection of the lung. A prolonged bout of pneumonia can cause severe ear infections, meningitis, and even death. Pneumonia is an extremely common infection. More than 150,000 cases are reported annually in the United States alone,[20] and more than one million children under five die worldwide each year as a result of the infection.[21] The two vaccines for pneumonia are the PCV13 and the PPSV23. Each vaccine carries an extremely rare risk of serious side effects.

Rotavirus is an infection that can cause dehydration. Nearly all Americans will catch rotavirus by their fifth birthday. More than fifty thousand babies are hospitalized because of rotavirus infection each year.[22] So, the risk of getting the disease is quite high. The initial vaccine was removed from the market because it was thought to increase a baby's risk of bowel intussusception. An intussusception is when the bowel telescopes back on itself and causes potentially serious problems. Since then, a new and improved vaccine is on the market with a far lower risk of side effects. The improved vaccine will prevent roughly 98 percent of all severe cases of rotavirus.[23] When balanced against the very high risk of infection and the low risk of side effects, the vaccine makes sense.

Rubella is an infection that has been largely eliminated in many countries as a result of vaccination. Most people who get rubella pass through the illness without even noticing it. Unfortunately, rubella infection can be quite harmful to fetuses. Infected fetuses are at great risk of serious side effects such as blindness and mental retardation. The vaccine is given with the measles and mumps antigens. It provides protection for pregnant women and their children. Severe reactions are estimated to be less than one in a million.[24]

Tetanus is a life-threatening illness that results from a bacterial infection. Tetanus cases are very rare. Fewer than one hundred people get sick each year.[25] However, this must be balanced against very high mortality rates should your child get infected. Tetanus is a very grave disease with a prolonged recovery period. The neonatal form of the disease kills thousands of babies in Africa annually. The tetanus vaccine is given with the vaccine for diphtheria and whooping cough. The vaccine provides protection against the disease for about ten years.[26] After that, health officials urge booster shots if you face a situation where you may be at risk. Since the tetanus vaccine is bundled with the diphtheria and pertussis vaccines into the DTaP, the risks of serious side effects from the vaccine are the same as for pertussis.

Whooping cough, or pertussis, is an extremely serious illness in babies and young children. A prolonged bout of whooping cough can easily lead to brain damage and even death in children under five. Whooping cough is a huge health problem both worldwide and in the United States. In recent years the number of pertussis cases has been rapidly on the rise. More than twenty-seven thousand cases were reported in 2010 in the United States alone.[27] The odds of a baby getting exposed to whooping cough are thus very high. The vaccine can be reactive and often leads to a mild reaction in many babies. The pertussis vaccine is traditionally bundled with antigens for diphtheria and tetanus. Moderate problems from the vaccine such as high fever can be as high as one in sixteen thousand vaccines.[28] When balanced against the possibility of getting such a serious illness, the odds still come out highly in favor of the vaccine.

THE VAERS DATABASE

Vaccines go through clinical trials before being brought to market. Once on the market vaccines are monitored in two ways. All vaccines in the United States go through a rigorous process of testing before they go into mass production for the general public. The second way that vaccines are monitored is long term through the VAERS database. The database is designed to help determine if a vaccine can cause side effects and to help victims establish a claim for aid if true.

The VAERS database is a collection of individual reports about vaccine reactions. The initials *VAERS* stand for Vaccine Adverse Event Reporting System. VAERS is a compilation of information about potential vaccine risks once the vaccine has come into widespread use by the public. The VAERS database is jointly sponsored by the Centers for Disease Control and Prevention and the Food and Drug Administration. The database relies on reporting by health professionals and the public. A person can fill out a report for database monitoring officials by mail, e-mail, or fax, or on the CDC website.

All reports follow the same format. The person reporting the event is asked to describe the sequence of events in as much detail as possible. Database administrators want to know information such as the time and date of the vaccine, where the vaccine was given, any preexisting conditions the recipient had as well as any medications the person is using, and any prior illnesses. Administrators are looking for extremely detailed information so they can narrow down potential risk factor that might make vaccine side effects more common in a given population.

Anyone can make a report to the database about any potential side effect after vaccination. A doctor can file a report about a rash he noticed on his patient's cheeks. A mom can write up an incident of fussiness after her daughter's second DTaP vaccination. Reports that lack details such as a child's birth weight or the specific vaccination lot are also accepted.

VAERS is completely accessible to the public. Anyone can comb through all filed reports online. The database is searchable by vaccine type and type of vaccine reaction such as fever. Database reports are periodically updated.

The VAERS database is intended to serve as a passive system. Health officials read every single report filed. If officials notice a pattern of specific reactions to a vaccine such as an increased number of cases of sudden infant death syndrome (SIDS) in the aftermath of a new vaccine, they will set up an investigation into the matter. Researchers want to determine if the result is a coincidence or a potential vaccine reaction.

If health officials notice a problem, further efforts are made to investigate it fully. A vaccine associated with even a small increased risk of side effects will be removed from the market. In 1999, officials removed the RotaShield vaccine from the market after finding a correlation between the vaccine and increased cases of intussusception of the bowel. That vaccine has since been replaced with a safer rotavirus vaccine.

The VAERS database is a useful tool when attempting to determine if a particular vaccine poses risks. Unfortunately, the database has serious flaws. The primary flaw of the database is that reports are not filtered. Raw data by itself means almost nothing. This is particularly true given the fact that anyone may file a report. Reports are not verified for accuracy unless health officials feel a pattern exists and further investigation is necessary. Individuals should be wary of examining the VAERS data and coming to a conclusion about a vaccine.

The database is also highly influenced by media or pop culture trends. At any given moment, a particular belief about specific vaccine side effects may be popular in the public mind. Lawyers seeking to capitalize on this perceived trend may encourage potential litigants to file reports on vaccine reactions to help bolster their arguments for more money from vaccine damage.

A report in the February 1, 2006, issue of *Pediatrics* highlights this problem. The authors found that the number of people reporting cases of alleged autism and vaccines can be correlated with the release in 1998 of the discredited study authored by Andrew Wakefield. Michael J. Goodman and James Nordin conclude, "The results of this article show a clear increase in VAERS reports related to litigation. Longitudinal analysis of adverse event reports that fail to take the reporting source into account will not portray accurately the trend that they imply in the data."[29] In other words, the database can be easily and deliberately manipulated by a group of individuals with an agenda. An informed parent must therefore approach the VAERS database with extreme caution.

IN SUMMARY: THE RISKS AND THE BENEFITS

Every single vaccine on the current American vaccine schedule carries at least some potential to cause a reaction. Your babies, toddlers, and children can never receive a shot without incurring some risks. The same is true of any given population including adolescents and seniors. Like just about every other activity you undertake, vaccination can never ever be truly free from risks. However, these risks are clearly balanced by two other risks: the risk of getting the disease and the risk that the disease can cause huge problems if you get sick.

Take diphtheria. Diphtheria cases are incredibly rare. Your family is at greater risk of getting struck by lightning or drowning in the bathtub than encountering a single case of diphtheria during their entire lives. Yet diphtheria has an enormous fatality rate and essentially no treatment. The vaccine has few risks and offers protection for life. The vaccine is coupled with the vaccines for tetanus and whooping cough, so your baby does not even need a separate series of shots to gain immunity.

A more common disease such as pertussis presents even better reason to choose vaccination. Pertussis is a nasty little illness that can literally turn your child blue from coughing and will most surely put your newborn in the hospital should she be so unlucky as to catch it. Pertussis is also on the rise, with thousands of cases annually. So the odds of your family coming into contact with someone with pertussis are fairly high. The biggest risk from the pertussis vaccine is not that the vaccine will cause a vaccine reaction. The biggest problem with the vaccine is that it will not work. This failure could leave your baby without protection should an outbreak occur. That's why doctors use multiple doses over a period of time.

The other vaccines on the typical vaccine schedule also have similar low risks and potentially high rewards. Many vaccine-preventable illnesses can be treated only with palliative measures. A pediatrician will give a child infected with measles more vitamin A, but that's only going to help reduce the effects of the illness and does not cure it. If your baby comes down with Hib, that baby will need to be closely watched in a pediatric hospital ward. A baby on a respirator as a result of whooping cough or who has a bad case of the flu may face months of painful recovery and hours of visits by medical professionals just to make sure he is finally okay even when he leaves the hospital. Teenagers who are sexually active have a one in two risk of getting HPV infection and putting themselves at greater risk for cancers of the reproductive system.[30] A 50 percent chance of becoming infected is a huge risk.

When you take on the slight risks of vaccination, you are also participating in a much larger and quite noble community effort. Vaccinated babies and children not only have protection for themselves but also help provide it for others.

Some babies and children cannot get vaccinated. A child who has specific allergies to ingredients in vaccines will be better off skipping certain individual vaccines. Children who are undergoing treatment for dangerous illnesses such as cancer often take medications that can compromise their immune systems. In that case, the vaccine may pose too great a risk to be used. Once in a while, a baby may have a very bad reaction to a vaccine. A pediatrician may advise against further use of a certain vaccine such as the DTaP. That does not mean your baby cannot get any other vaccines at all. It just means your baby may be a little too sensitive to the antigen in the pertussis vaccine. If this happens, your baby relies on others for protection.

If your child is one of those who cannot be vaccinated for any of these reasons, the best possible course of action you can take is to advocate vaccination for others. The only protection your child will have against an outbreak of measles or whooping cough or the flu is people who have been vaccinated. Their decision to vaccinate forms the only safety net your unvaccinated child will ever have. Punching holes in this net by actively encouraging nonvaccination only serves to increase your child's medical risks.

A close look at the risks reveals a simple calculus. People should vaccinate their children for many important reasons. Vaccination not only offers protection from many diseases at low personal risk but also reduces the severity of most diseases should your child get sick. Vaccination also offers an additional benefit. When you vaccinate your child, you're also helping to build a ring of protection around your entire community. The little girl with leukemia who cannot get vaccinated, the young boy who reacts badly to the whooping cough vaccine, the kidney transplant patient—all reduce their odds of getting a vaccine-preventable disease when you and your family show up for well-baby visits.

Your vaccinated children are their only form of protection.

· 7 ·

Vaccines and Autism:
The Creation of a Modern Myth

$\mathcal{I}$n 1998, the highly respected British medical journal *The Lancet* published a study that claimed to find a link between the measles, mumps,
and rubella (MMR) vaccine and the symptoms of autism in children.[1] The
story was immediately picked up and sensationalized by the British and
international media.

Twelve years later, *The Lancet* retracted publication of that study. Such
a retraction in effect is an admission that the article should never have been
published in the first place.[2]

What happened in between those two dates involves hysteria, finger-
pointing, fearmongering, and a widespread and growing effort to deliberately
mislead the public about the supposed link between vaccines and autism.

This supposed link is probably the number one reason parents express
hesitation about vaccinating their children. In 2011 in Colorado, parents continued to cite this study as justification for their suspicion of vaccines.[3] Let's
take the study and walk through it step by step.

THE LANCET STUDY—
WIDELY MISREAD AND NOT READ AT ALL

Although *The Lancet* retracted the study discussed here, the original text
(with the large red "RETRACTED" superimposed upon it) is still available
at *The Lancet*'s website. We encourage you to read it yourself. Surprisingly,
it's quite short.

The original study involved a group of thirteen coauthors, headed by Dr. Andrew Wakefield. Wakefield was a British gastroenterologist, a surgeon specializing in the treatment of issues of the digestive tract. He was conducting research into Crohn's disease, a digestive disorder, when a woman whose son had been diagnosed with autism and digestive issues contacted him. He claims she convinced him to conduct research into a possible link between autism and digestive disorders.

Wakefield and his coauthors studied twelve children, eleven boys and one girl. All of them were being treated for digestive issues at a pediatric gastroenterologist clinic. In addition, all of them had been developmentally normal but had lost developmental milestones such as speech. Nine of the children had been diagnosed with autism. One of the children had been diagnosed with disintegrative psychosis, and two had been diagnosed with encephalitis. The study claimed to find a link between all of these diagnoses and the children's digestive issues. The authors claimed to have identified a never-before-seen condition that they called autistic enterocolitis. They stated that the onset of the condition had been reported by the parents to be associated with the children's receiving the MMR vaccine.

The authors claimed to have found consistent abnormalities in the digestive tracts of the children (hence their treatment at a specialty clinic) but inconsistencies in the onset of the behavioral and developmental symptoms. Some of the children had shown very rapid decline, while others had shown slower signs of deterioration. Some of the children had classic symptoms of a Pervasive Developmental Disorder, while others showed signs of other disorders.

The original article specifically states, "We did not prove an association with the measles, mumps and rubella vaccine and the syndrome described."[4]

Let us repeat that statement, because it is crucial. The authors of the original piece of research that is the supposed smoking gun regarding the link between vaccines and autism state in their very own article, "We did not prove an association with the measles, mumps, and rubella vaccine and the syndrome described."[4]

In spite of their own statement that an association between the MMR vaccine and autism was not proven, the authors go on to say that more research is needed to continue to investigate the possibility of a link between the MMR vaccine and autism. And actually, we agree. We agreed then, and we would agree now, if the study were published now. A small study like this that seems to show some preliminary results should absolutely be followed up by further research to investigate the possible link. Such follow-up research has been performed, on multiple continents, with multiple research groups both privately and government funded, using multiple research designs. All of that research has actually replicated the original result of the Wakefield study—no link between vaccines and autism has been found.

The issue isn't with the original study's conclusions as they are written. The issue is with what the authors, specifically Andrew Wakefield, did with the study's conclusions. The issue is also with what the media did with the study's result. As a direct result of the media frenzy and Wakefield's continued support of his supposed findings, thirteen years later there are needless epidemics of childhood diseases in many parts of the developed world.

Andrew Wakefield, upon the publication of this original article in *The Lancet*, called a press conference and released a video. In that video, he made the startling, and unsupported, statement that his research had raised a question about the safety of the MMR vaccine. He further stated that as a physician, he could not support the continued use of the vaccine. In spite of his own research stating that a link between the MMR vaccine and the disorders seen in the subjects had not been proven, he went on record as stating that the research supported not using the vaccine anymore. He claims instead that using three different vaccines (measles, mumps, and rubella) instead of the composite one was the logical outcome of his research. He did not give any reason for the differences between his public statements and his own published research findings.

Thus began the media storm of inaccurate reporting of the research findings, and the resulting anti-vaccine panic, to this date, has resulted in a resurgence of previously controlled childhood infectious diseases. Children have died of vaccine-preventable diseases in the years since Wakefield's study was released to the public.

THE STUDY—STEP BY STEP

Small Sample Size

The first thing we need to look at is Wakefield's subjects. In research, a general rule is that the larger the sample size, the more the results apply to the rest of the population. This is known as generalizability. However, small sample sizes are often used in what are called pilot studies, when researchers test out their original research design to see if any unforeseen flaws appear. So, the fact that the original research included only twelve children, eleven of whom were boys, is not in and of itself a red flag that the research is invalid.

However, in small sample sizes, odd results will sometimes appear. You may have heard of the Mozart effect. The Mozart effect refers to a study that supposedly found that playing classical music to your children makes them smarter. In the Mozart effect study, researchers had thirty-six college students listen to classical music, a relaxation tape, and nothing for ten minutes before taking some spatial reasoning tests that are part of the traditional Stanford-Binet intelligence test. The researchers noted that in the classical music situation, the scores were higher than in the relaxation tape condition or the silence condition.

When a study uses a small number of people, you often end up with results that are not found when you repeat the research with larger groups of people. Repeating research using larger or more varied groups of subjects is a process called replication. This process is vital for determining the validity of scientific research results. Attempts to replicate the results of the original Mozart study have been inconsistent.

Obviously, people who are interested in the link between the MMR vaccine and autism (even though the original study specifically stated that such a link was not proven) will want to replicate the research. They'll want to do so using more subjects. And they have. We'll discuss those studies shortly.

How the Subjects Were Chosen

The second thing we want to look at is Wakefield's sampling strategy. In scientific research, a valid research sample is one that's chosen via random sampling—every person in the group being studied has an equal chance of being chosen for participation. In the Wakefield study, the group that was the focus of the research were children who had a history of (1) digestive disorders, (2) diagnoses of autism, and (3) reports by their parents that the developmental regression began shortly after the children received the MMR vaccine.

If you're a scientist, you'll want to figure out the relationship between all of those variables. In order to do so, you might want to *start* with children who have all of those variables in common. But if you do that, you've basically designed a case study. You've chosen people in a biased fashion, not randomly. You've deliberately picked them out because they display the variables in which you're interested. Wakefield started out studying whether or not there was a relationship between digestive disorders, autism, and reports of MMR vaccine exposure by deliberately choosing to study *only* those children who met that criteria.

Case studies are great places to start out. They generate questions for future study. They provide illustrative cases for already established relationships. But information gathered in case studies cannot be applied to the rest of the population. The sampling for case studies is biased, and the sample sizes are too small.

Therefore, the original study was valuable as a starting point. That starting point did not find a relationship between the MMR vaccine and autism but proposed that further research was needed. In spite of the lack of any significant finding, the lead author, Andrew Wakefield, went on record to state that the MMR vaccine was dangerous and, in his opinion, should not be used. This statement was in direct contradiction to the findings of his own research.

The media bears some responsibility in this fiasco. Most journalists are not trained in a scientific field or in the scientific method. Therefore, they tend to misunderstand or misinterpret research data as it is presented. Most people who read the newspaper or the Internet or watch television news are similarly untrained. They are likely to hear the media reports of research and accept them at face value. Only a very, very small percentage of the general public might spend the actual time and effort to go back to the original study the media is covering and read that study for themselves. In this particular case, that natural tendency to believe the media has had significantly negative consequences ever since.

What Was Studied

Let's look at the variables investigated in the Wakefield study. The original study was designed to investigate a link between digestive disorders and Pervasive Developmental Disorders in children. In addition, the symptoms of those disorders had supposedly appeared (according to their parents' reports) relatively soon after those children had received MMR vaccines. So, if you're going to investigate those variables, you'll want to make sure of the following:

1. That the digestive disorders existed independently of the parents' observations (in other words, the parents were not the only people who observed digestive disorders in the children)
2. That the Pervasive Developmental Disorders existed independently of the parents' observations and were diagnosed by professionals in the field of child psychopathology (the field that specializes in childhood psychological or behavioral disorders)
3. The vaccination schedule, status, and dates of the children involved
4. That vaccinations had indeed predated either the digestive disorders or the Pervasive Developmental Disorder symptoms or both
5. That no symptoms of digestive disorders or Pervasive Developmental Disorders were observed either by parents or by professionals before the vaccines were administered

In the original study, the subjects had been diagnosed with digestive disorders and were being treated at a pediatric specialty clinic for children with digestive issues. The Pervasive Development Disorder symptoms were reported by parents, and the children's psychiatric diagnoses had been made elsewhere.

Lack of Verification

There is no evidence in the original *Lancet* article that children received the MMR vaccine prior to the onset of either their digestive disorders or their diagnosis of any developmental disorders. The parents reported that the children's vaccines had preceded the problems, but the authors do not report verifying these statements. Indeed, the authors did not report that they had verified the parents had had their children vaccinated at all. This may seem as if it is a small issue. But, this was a study in which the relationship between vaccines and other symptoms was one of the main relationships being investigated. Why wouldn't the researchers have verified through medical records that the children had received the vaccines their parents had reported?

You may think this statement calls parents liars. That is certainly not our intent. In scientific research, secondhand reports that can be verified *must* be verified. People's memories are fallible—people forget dates, times, events. If written records exist to verify verbal reports, it is the duty of scientists to use those written reports. There is no evidence that the study's authors did so in terms of the reports of vaccines received.

Lack of Consistent Temporal Relationships

The reported onset of behavioral symptoms leading to the diagnosis of autism or other Pervasive Developmental Disorders was anywhere from twenty-four hours to two *months* after the children allegedly received the vaccine. There was no consistent pattern of timing between the supposed receipt of the vaccine and when the children began displaying the symptoms that led to their diagnosis. In fact, one of the subjects was reportedly developing normally until about fifteen months of age. Then, that subject underwent a slowing of development but didn't experience a sudden loss of developed skills until four or five years of age!

This lack of a consistent relationship between the time of a vaccine and the time of the symptoms' appearance greatly undermines Wakefield's original study. This weakness is also found in any other research that claims to find a relationship between vaccines and disorders such as autism. Some parents claimed to see an immediate loss of skills (speech, movement, social interaction, and so on) the *second* their child received a vaccine. Other parents claimed to see a gradual loss of those skills over the course of days or weeks after a vaccine. This lack of a consistent pattern is more likely to be explained by factors other than vaccines. This lack of a temporal pattern should have been mentioned in the original study. It was not.

There are a couple of factors to consider when parents report changes in their children's developmental milestones. First, some parents have a tendency to overlook early symptoms of Pervasive Developmental Disorders such as autism. The characteristic lack of social interest or social interaction in children with autism might be seen in infants and simply put down to temperamental differences, or shyness, or other factors. In one case that Allison had personal experience with, the parents were originally concerned that their child was deaf or suffered some hearing delays. It was only at Allison's urging that the parents obtained professional assessment that led to the diagnosis of autism. Prior to that assessment, the parents simply kept taking their child in for hearing tests.

Second, development is not linear. Children may progress in reaching developmental milestones and then regress and lose those milestones for a myriad of reasons or for no clear discernible reason at all. The gaining of developmental milestones, the lack of that gain, the gain and then the loss—all are part of both normal development and of pathological development. When this natural ebb and flow of development is complicated by real conditions, parents naturally look around for some process that is responsible for any change. Receiving a vaccine is often scary for the child, with the result that the child cries or expresses much unhappiness and discomfort. Some reactions to vaccines are normal but unexpected. It's easy for the parents to latch onto the vaccine as the source of the developmental change.

Lack of Consistent Digestive Findings

The Wakefield study did find that all of the children had specific problems in several measures of their digestive function, but that was expected since all the children were receiving specialized treatment for that issue. However, there was not a consistent pattern of digestive issues in relation to the onset of behavior symptoms *or* to receiving the MMR vaccine. Some of the children began experiencing digestive problems around the same time they began showing behavioral issues. Other children showed digestive issues prior to the behavioral symptoms. Still others showed digestive issues only after the behavioral issues showed up. In half the children in the study, the date of onset of the digestive issues was reported as unknown. That latter statistic is especially troubling in a study designed to investigate any relationship between vaccines, digestive issues, and the diagnosis of autism.

Lack of Measles Virus

A key issue in trying to find a relationship between the MMR vaccine, digestive disorders, and autism would involve finding traces of the vaccine virus in the tissues of the children involved. Viruses used in vaccines are often different from wild viruses—sometimes vaccines use an attenuated version of the wild virus, and sometimes vaccines use a killed version of the wild virus. Researchers who were interested in finding a link between the virus in a vaccine and symptoms in the person receiving the vaccine would want to find traces of the vaccine-type virus in the subjects, right? Except that Wakefield and his fellow researchers did not find those traces. The tissues of the subjects in their 1998 research did not contain the measles vaccine virus. Without that, any attempt to link symptoms to the vaccine is definitely not supported by the data from the research study.

The Study's Conclusions

The final paragraph of the Wakefield study is included here so you can see for yourself some of the issues in their statements:

> We have identified a chronic enterocolitis in children that may be related to neuropsychiatric dysfunction. In most cases, onset of symptoms was after measles, mumps, and rubella immunization [*sic*]. Further investigations are needed to examine this syndrome and its possible relation to this vaccine.[5]

Note that the very first sentence of that concluding paragraph cannot be supported by the study's own data. The digestive issues seen in the children could not be consistently linked to the neuropsychiatric dysfunction. The phrase *neuropsychiatric dysfunction* in this case means the diagnoses of autism or other Pervasive Developmental Disorders. The pattern of onset of digestive issues was not consistently related to the pattern of onset of behavioral issues. The second sentence of that concluding paragraph also cannot be supported by the study's own data. The onset of either the digestive or the behavioral symptoms could not be consistently related to the children's receiving the MMR vaccine. The only reasonable sentence in that paragraph is the third sentence. Further study should be done, given the small sample size of this original study.

As you can see, the original source of the media-driven myth that vaccines cause autism actually does not support that conclusion *at all*. If that is the case, then why was and is the world convinced of such a link? That can be traced to the behavior of the lead author, Andrew Wakefield, after the publication of the article.

ANDREW WAKEFIELD —
MISREPRESENTING HIS OWN STUDY

After *The Lancet* published the study, Wakefield held a press conference[6] and released several video and print press releases. In those communications to the media, he firmly stated that in his professional and research opinion, the MMR vaccine was too dangerous to continue to be administered to children. He encouraged British society to remain cautious about the use of this vaccine, citing his own study. As we have seen, the study did not prove anything of the kind.

That did not stop the British media, and soon the international media, from latching onto the story. The media spread fear of the vaccine throughout the developed world. Reporters are not scientists. In many cases, they do not even read the studies they are writing about. Guided by Wakefield, the media hammered the medical community for continuing to support the use of such a dangerous vaccine. As a result of this coverage, vaccine rates began to fall in Britain and elsewhere. Within a few years, measles vaccine rates in Britain had dropped below 85 percent. For a population to have herd immunity against measles, the vaccine rate must be at least 83 percent. Some estimates place that needed percentage as high as 92 percent.[7] As vaccine rates fell in the aftermath of the Wakefield publicity, measles rates began to climb in Britain. In 1998, during the beginning of the onslaught of media publicity, Britain experienced fifty-six cases of measles. In the first five months of 2006, there were 449 cases. The numbers have continued to fluctuate but have never dropped to the low levels seen prior to the Wakefield scare.

At no time did Wakefield correct the press reports claiming a link between the MMR vaccine and autism. He allowed these reports to continue even though they were not supported by his own findings. Indeed, he actively participated in the ongoing spread of inaccurate data and freely participated in the attacks on the medical community. He continued to insist that children should not receive the MMR vaccine because it increased their chances of developing autism. He encouraged parents to demand that those three vaccines be given separately, rather than in a combined dose, and continued to rail against the MMR vaccine, implicitly encouraging a public fear of the MMR vaccine in particular and of vaccines in general. He was the only one of the original thirteen authors to do so in such a public fashion. To this day, parents who are reluctant to vaccinate their children cite Wakefield as the prime reason for their fears.

CONCERNS ABOUT WAKEFIELD

Soon after the publication of the Wakefield study and the media storm that followed, questions began to arise in the British medical community about the study and about the lead author. He and another research team had produced earlier research in 1994 that claimed to find a link between the measles virus and/or the measles vaccine and the digestive disorder Crohn's disease.[8] The results of that earlier piece of research, like the 1998 research, have never been replicated by other researchers.[9] Because of Wakefield's history of presenting research results that other scientists could not repeat, people started asking questions. They found some interesting information.

In 1997, Wakefield filed a request for a grant of patent for a vaccine he had designed to be a substitute or replacement for the MMR vaccine currently in use in Britain at that time.[10] He filed the patent application in 1998.[11] This patent application was not revealed to the editorial board of *The Lancet* at the time of the original publication of Wakefield's article. His partner in the patent was a gentleman named Herman Hugh Fudenberg (listed as "Fundenberg" on the patent application). Dr. Fudenberg is a South Carolina doctor whose license was suspended in 1995, after the South Carolina medical board found him "guilty of engaging in dishonorable, unethical, or unprofessional conduct." His license to practice completely expired in 2004.[12,13] He does not currently hold a medical license. Dr. Fudenberg has claimed to be able to cure autism by using his own bone marrow, which he prepared in his home kitchen.[14] He also claims there is a link between the flu shot and Alzheimer's disease. No scientific evidence supports these claims.[15]

In 2004, the London *Sunday Times* published an article that revealed that Wakefield's study was funded in part by a consortium of lawyers. The lawyers had recruited doctors and scientists to engage in research designed to "prove" that the MMR vaccine was unsafe. Wakefield received more than 430,000 British pounds (approximately $688,000) from this group of lawyers. The lawyers had been hired by a group of parents who claimed their children had been harmed in some way by the MMR vaccine. Ethical researchers are expected to reveal their funding sources to not only their co-authors but also the editorial board of the publication that is publishing the study. Wakefield did not reveal this source of funding to *The Lancet*. The same consortium of lawyers gave money to Wakefield's business partners and the experts he used in his research.[16]

Also in 2004, ten of Wakefield's twelve original coauthors retracted their support of the study's conclusions. Their retraction repeated the original paper's findings that no causal link between the MMR vaccine and autism was found. The coauthors stated they were withdrawing their interpretation of the original data because of the profound negative effect the proposed link was having on the public welfare of Britain. They specifically cited the declining MMR vaccination rates as one of the reasons for their retraction.[17]

Over the years since 2004, more has come to light about Wakefield's background and credentials. This information gives us some possible motives he may have had for misrepresenting the results of his own research.

Some of the parents of the children in Wakefield's study claim that the symptoms reported in the study do not match the symptoms their children were actually exhibiting. These parents provided medical records that do indeed reflect discrepancies between the symptoms the children were exhibiting and the symptoms Wakefield claimed they were exhibiting. There were already concerns about the symptoms and diagnoses discussed in the study, and this revelation provided more.[18]

Some of the parents dispute the timeline that Wakefield listed with regard to the onset of behavior symptoms and the timing of the children's MMR vaccine. Those parents confirmed that their children had actually begun exhibiting symptoms prior to the vaccine. Their children were reported in the study as having received the vaccine and then starting to display symptoms.[18]

The children were described in the study as having regressive autism. This is a term used to indicate that the children were developmentally normal until a certain point, at which point they regressed, or lost their skills. This type of autism is different from the classic autism symptoms that are present and identified early. However, only one of the children in the study actually had regressive autism, and three of the other children had no diagnosis of autism at all.[18]

Some of the children in the study had digestive issues prior to their receipt of the MMR vaccine. The study attempted to determine whether the digestive issues were related to autism and whether both were caused by the MMR vaccine. If digestive issues occurred prior to the administration of the MMR vaccine, clearly no causal link between the two can be assumed.[18]

The children had biopsies performed on their digestive tracts. The resulting tissue samples were sent for analysis. The initial pathology reports on the tissues did not find any indication of pathologies. Only when those samples were sent to one of the coauthor's labs did any of the tests indicate physical pathologies. That coauthor, incidentally, is not one of the ten who retracted support of the study.[18]

There are other concerns not connected to the 1998 article. At his son's birthday party in 1999, Wakefield paid children at the party five British pounds each to allow him to draw their blood for testing. He drew those blood samples right there at the party. He did not have any institutional or research board approval to engage in this behavior. He later publicly joked about the incident, claiming he intended to continue gathering study samples in this way.[19] Obviously, this behavior in no way meets the ethical or scientific expectations of appropriate researcher behavior.

In 2007, the General Medical Council (GMC) began an investigation into the case. The GMC is the United Kingdom's regulatory body that oversees doctors. It specifically focused on Wakefield and two coauthors—John Angus Walker-Smith and Simon Murch. The GMC maintains a registry of practitioners allowed to practice medicine in the United Kingdom. It also can restrict doctors from practicing.

The GMC investigation into Wakefield, Walker-Smith, and Murch lasted almost three years. The panel interviewed thirty-six witnesses in addition to the three doctors under investigation. They spent forty-five days deliberating on the evidence that had been gathered. At the end of that time, the three were found to have been guilty of unethical, irresponsible, and dishonest conduct.[20] The GMC then stripped both Wakefield and Walker-Smith of their medical credentials, a process known as "struck off." This means that Andrew Wakefield, the person who is directly responsible for the perpetuation of the myth that vaccines cause autism, has had his medical licensure revoked in Britain. He is no longer allowed to practice medicine in that country. As he does not possess an American medical license, he also cannot practice medicine in the United States. Dr. Walker-Smith appealed the GMC's decision and won his appeal in 2012.

THE AFTERMATH—THE DAMAGE AND THE CONTINUING MYTH

Andrew Wakefield's conduct might not have been a problem if his claimed research results (which his own study contradicted) had proven to be valid and reliable. If other researchers, building on his small study, had been able to repeat his results, the information would have been of extreme importance. Our understanding of the benefits and disadvantages of vaccines would have been fundamentally altered. There would be very different recommendations in place in terms of what vaccines are recommended and when. We'd also be much closer to an understanding of what causes autism, which remains a troubling and baffling diagnosis.

We are none of those things. Multiple studies in multiple countries over multiple years have been unable to locate any link between the MMR vaccine and autism or any other vaccines and autism.

Wakefield continues to claim that such a link exists. He calls himself a victim of a conspiracy between the medical establishment and pharmaceutical companies. He gives presentations in which he attacks vaccines, the World Health Organization, the Centers for Disease Control and Prevention, and anyone else he can think of. He accuses them of covering up a vast, worldwide, multidecade conspiracy to use vaccines to harm children and to hide the dangers of vaccines. He insists that none of the named issues were true, or that they were misinterpreted, or that his conduct was taken out of context, or that there are perfectly reasonable explanations for the issues that were found.[21]

And in the meantime, vaccine rates for measles, mumps, rubella, chicken pox, and whooping cough remain below those necessary for herd immunity. Worse, children are dying of diseases that until recently were unlikely to kill.

Autism: A Brief Discussion of the Facts

"*Y*our child has autism."

That's a very frightening statement for a parent to hear. It's made more frightening by the fact that scientists still do not understand the cause of autism. But we do know this—the scientific consensus is that vaccines are not related to autism. The research studies simply do not support that belief. Over the years, there have been dozens of studies with hundreds of thousands of subjects, looking at a wide variety of vaccine-related issues. Some of those studies have looked at thimerosal and other ingredients in vaccines. Others have looked at the vaccines themselves. None have replicated Andrew Wakefield's supposed link between vaccines and autism.

THIMEROSAL STUDIES

One of the claims made by the anti-vaccine movement is that the thimerosal preservative in vaccines is the substance that causes autism. Thimerosal metabolizes in the body into ethylmercury. Since methylmercury has been found to be poisonous to brain and nerve cells, people assumed that ethylmercury was toxic. Therefore, much of the early anti-vaccine movement focused on this particular substance. Let's look at the studies about this issue.

In Denmark, a group of researchers analyzed medical records about the relationship between psychiatric treatment and vaccines. Danish children received diphtheria, tetanus, and pertussis (DTaP) vaccines containing thimerosal from 1961 to 1970. From 1970 to 1992, thimerosal was found in the stand-alone pertussis vaccine. After 1992, vaccines in Denmark no longer contained thimerosal. If thimerosal was a culprit in the onset of autism, removing it would be expected to result in a decrease in autism rates. The research group looked at all psychiatric admissions to Danish hospitals from 1971 to 2000 and all outpatient psychiatric department contacts from 1995 to 2000. They correlated the diagnoses of autism with the amount of thimerosal received by the children with those diagnoses. They found that the incidence of autism did not decrease after Danish children stopped being exposed to thimerosal in the vaccine schedule. Instead, the researchers found that the number of children diagnosed with autism *increased* after 1992.[1]

Similarly, a group of British researchers analyzed the records of 107,152 children born between 1988 and 1997. They compiled vaccination histories to determine the amount of thimerosal the children had received throughout their childhood. The researchers then looked at any diagnoses in medical records. They found no correlation between the amount of thimerosal the children were exposed to and any neurological diagnoses, including autism. Indeed, they, too, found that the incidence of diagnoses of certain disorders was slightly *higher* for children who'd received fewer thimerosal-containing vaccines.[2]

In 2004, a group of researchers, including ones from the Centers for Disease Control and Prevention (CDC) in Atlanta, analyzed twelve studies. All of these studies looked at a possible link between thimerosal and autistic spectrum disorders, or ASDs (autism, Asperger's syndrome, and Pervasive Developmental Disorder Not Otherwise Specified). This type of review is called a meta-analysis. It is a good way for outside researchers to take a look at a lot of studies that all covered the same ground. The reviewers can then pull the scientifically valid results together to look for patterns. The researchers in the 2004 meta-analysis looked at ten studies comparing rates of the disorders and the presence of thimerosal in vaccines. These types of studies are known as epidemiological studies. The other two studies were pharmacokinetic, meaning those studies looked at the levels of thimerosal in the body after children received vaccines containing the substance.

The 2004 meta-analysis found that four studies supported an association between thimerosal and ASDs. All four of those studies were performed by the same research team, a father and son named Mark and David Geier. The data and their research are considered too methodologically flawed to be considered valid. The remaining eight scientifically valid studies indicated no evidence of a link between the presence of thimerosal in vaccines and the rates of diagnosis of ASDs. Those studies also did not find a link between the amount of thimerosal received in a vaccine history and the rates of diagnosis of ASDs.[3]

In 2008, researchers wanted to see if the body processed ethylmercury and methylmercury differently. They looked at the amount of thimerosal in an infant's body after the child receives a vaccine. Thimerosal has been removed from all childhood vaccines in the United States, with the exception of some flu vaccines. Therefore, the researchers looked at 216 infants in Argentina, where thimerosal is still found in childhood vaccines. They found that the type of mercury in thimerosal (ethylmercury) stays in the body for much, much less time than methylmercury, which is the type of mercury found in fish or in pollution. Ethylmercury had a half-life of 3.7 days, while methylmercury had a half-life of 44 days. Half-life is the amount of time it takes for the body to process half of the substance. Until this study, it was assumed that both types of mercury would stay in the body for the same amount of time. However, the ethylmercury in thimerosal is processed out of the body too quickly to build up to the toxic levels claimed by the anti-vaccine movement. Fundamentally, the fearmongering about mercury being toxic in the body is based on information regarding a completely different type of mercury![4]

Thimerosal was discontinued in Canadian vaccines in 1996. In 2006, Canadian researchers surveyed 27,749 children who were born from 1987 to 1998. They compared diagnoses of Pervasive Developmental Disorders between the children who received vaccines containing thimerosal and the children who did not. Ironically, the researchers found a significant *increase* in the prevalence rates of Pervasive Developmental Disorders in the children who had received the thimerosal-free vaccines. They also found that rates of diagnosis of Pervasive Developmental Disorder did not change after Canadian doctors introduced, in 1996, a vaccine schedule that included a second measles, mumps, and rubella (MMR) dose. The rates were the same whether the children received one MMR vaccine or two MMR vaccines.[5]

These are but a few of the many studies that have investigated any link between thimerosal and autism and have found nothing. Unfortunately, these studies aren't enough for the anti-vaccine movement. After thimerosal was ruled out as a causal factor, the anti-vaccine movement began to claim that the vaccines themselves were dangerous. Scientists responded to these claims as scientists always do, by studying the new proposed links. This is the nature of research—as new possible hypotheses present themselves, scientists explore those through new research.

STUDIES OF VACCINES WITHOUT THIMEROSAL

Finnish researchers investigated a possible link between the MMR vaccine, gastrointestinal disorders, and autism. This is the same link that Wakefield claimed to study. They followed children for sixteen years, from 1982 to 1998. They tracked the vaccine schedules of those children and any development of either digestive disorders or autism. Their research ended up including three million vaccine doses. Thirty-one children were reported as developing gastrointestinal problems after receiving the MMR vaccine. None of those children developed autism or other Pervasive Developmental Disorders, and the gastrointestinal problems were not linked to the vaccine.[6]

British researchers identified 498 children born since 1979 who had different types of autism. The researchers looked at the temporal relationship between those children's symptoms and their vaccination histories. The MMR vaccine was introduced in Britain in 1988. There was not a sudden spike of autism cases after that date. There was a steady increase in the rates of diagnosis over the years. Some of the children had received the vaccine before eighteen months of age, and others had received the vaccine after that age. Some of the children had never been vaccinated at all. There was no difference in the rates of diagnosis of autism in the three groups of children.[7]

Danish researchers looked at the vaccination records of all children born in Denmark between January 1991 and December 1998. They were able to obtain medical records for a total of 537,303 children. Remember that the Wakefield study looked at only twelve children. Of the Danish group, 440,665 children received the MMR vaccine. There was no difference in the rates of autism between the children who received the vaccine and the children who did not.[8]

In 2008, researchers attempted to perform a critical scientific task—finding the same results as Andrew Wakefield originally claimed. This process of replication is vital in the scientific method, especially when results are from such small studies as Wakefield's. The 2008 researchers, like Wakefield et al., studied the relationship between gastrointestinal disturbances, autism, and the receipt of the MMR vaccine. They studied twenty-five children with both autism and gastrointestinal issues and compared them to thirteen children with gastrointestinal issues but without any diagnosis of autism (the control group). They followed the steps reported in the original Wakefield article in terms of the tests performed and the validation of the diagnoses. These researchers were unable to replicate Wakefield's supposed results—in other words, they did not find a temporal link between the MMR vaccine, the onset of gastrointestinal problems, and the onset of autism symptoms.[9]

This chapter could go on and on and on, listing and discussing the huge number of studies that have continually found no link between the MMR vaccine without thimerosal and autism, and between vaccines in general and autism. Rather than waste your time, we have simply listed them in the notes section for this chapter so you can read them on your own. Most of them are available with full text online so you can see for yourself what we are reporting. These studies were performed in many different countries

(Japan,[10] the United States,[11] Canada,[5,12] Denmark,[13] the United Kingdom). They were performed by researchers from many different institutions and groups (universities, hospitals, government agencies). They looked at many different variables—the presence or absence of virus antibodies in the bodies of children, the timing of the vaccines, the types of vaccine schedules. They measured their variables in many different ways. All of the research designs were methodologically sound and valid. None of them have been retracted or found to be flawed, fraudulent, or biased. And the overwhelming pattern of results indicates no link between vaccines and autism.

WHY DO PEOPLE INSIST THERE IS A LINK BETWEEN VACCINES AND AUTISM?

There's a simple explanation of why people continue to believe in a disproved link. Cognitive biases.

Humans naturally look for patterns in the world around them. The tendency to identify a relationship between two variables and maintain a belief in that relationship can be explained using cognitive psychology. What a person remembers is often unusual or vivid in some way. That event or piece of information stands out from the background of the person's ordinary life. Anything that stands out becomes easier to remember. This is called the availability heuristic. What's vivid becomes available in our memories.

Once we've remembered the vivid event, we tend to associate other things with that event. We break a leg, and we remember things around that event. Our baby cries with a vaccine reaction, and we remember things we noticed happening at that time. We build a belief that those two things are related. This belief may not be supported by research, but that doesn't matter to our non-scientific minds. We maintain a belief in the relationship between those two variables in spite of a lack of evidence. This is known as an illusory correlation.

After an illusory correlation is established, we keep it going through the confirmation bias. The confirmation bias is our natural tendency to seek out or notice information that confirms our preexisting belief system. In other words, we see the times when the world tells us we are right. Conversely, we also ignore or actively reject times when the world tells us we are wrong. If we believe our child's problems are related to vaccines, we'll notice or remember all the problems we noticed after the vaccine but ignore or forget any problems we noticed before the vaccine.

We then also start to notice reports of other children having vaccine reactions. What goes unrecognized are all the instances in which children receiving vaccines are not diagnosed with autism, or the instances in which children not receiving vaccines are diagnosed with autism.

All of these mean parents are likely to remember their children's vaccine reactions if those reactions are vivid or unusual. They are then likely to remember their children's behavior around that time and pay attention to unusual or worrying behavior. Then, they believe the vaccines and the behavior are related. They remember behavior that occurred after the vaccines and not behavior that occurred prior to the vaccines. Finally, they begin to notice similar reports from other parents, strengthening their belief that vaccines are related to (and cause) children's developmental problems.

IF VACCINES DON'T CAUSE AUTISM, WHAT DOES?

We don't know. That's the short and unpleasant answer.

How can we not know by now? Because autism, and the other ASDs, are complicated syndromes. There are multiple areas and possible causes to research. Some of that research requires more time so researchers can follow the developmental progress of children for years in order to track contributing factors. Some of the research is complicated by the fact that scarce research dollars keep getting diverted to other areas of study, such as continuing to study the disproven links between vaccines and autism.

We do know there is a genetic component, since autism runs in families. Multiple variations in genetic codes have been identified.[14] Some of those variations in genetics appear to be inherited, while others appear to be random mutations. Since multiple genes have been implicated, it's difficult for researchers to narrow their focus. In addition, how those genetic variations contribute to autism is still a mystery.[15,16,17]

There are biological factors involved as well. Some research has found that the spacing of pregnancies is associated with an increased likelihood of a diagnosis of autism. Children born shortly after a firstborn sibling were at an increased risk of developing autism, with the highest risk being found in pregnancies that were less than one year apart.[18] Maternal and paternal age is associated with autism, with older ages related to an increased likelihood of autism.[19] Parents of children diagnosed with autism are more likely to have a history of psychiatric disorders.[20] Mothers with certain infections during pregnancy are more likely to have children who are diagnosed with autism.[21]

There appear to be some physical factors associated with autism as well. We know that autism is associated with an increased number of neurons in the prefrontal cortex.[22] In addition, very early preterm infants were more likely to exhibit autism-like behaviors,[23] possibly due to cerebral hemorrhagic injury.[24] The hippocampus is enlarged in children and adolescents with autism.[25]

The bottom line is there are multiple lines of research into the causes of autism.[26,27] So far, it appears there are genetic, biological, viral, and possibly environmental factors that contribute to the development of autism spectrum disorders. But regardless of the complexity of the causes, the research indicates that autism is not related to vaccines, whether they contain thimerosal or not.

THEN WHY ARE THE RATES OF AUTISM GOING UP?

First, we have to talk about what autism actually is. Autism is part of a broader category of childhood illnesses called Pervasive Developmental Disorders (PDDs). Other types of PDDs are Asperger's syndrome, Childhood Disintegrative Disorder, Rett syndrome, and PDD Not Otherwise Specified (PDD-NOS). The last condition is a catch-all diagnosis that's used when a child has some form of PDD but doesn't clearly fall into any of the disorders.

Autism is a developmental disorder that affects a wide variety of behaviors and mental processes. In the classic, traditional presentation of autism, the child may never learn to speak or communicate with others. In milder cases, some communication is possible, but that communication may be limited or highly idiosyncratic. Some children exhibit ritualized, repetitive behaviors, such as rocking back and forth, waving or flapping their hands, or spinning in circles. Children with autism may develop obsessive fixations on subjects, spending all of their waking time talking, studying, and learning about that subject. They may spend hours with one single object—a toy, for example. They have trouble with social interactions—they struggle with eye contact or with give-and-take conversations. They misread, ignore, or miss obvious social cues from others, such as if another child walks away after a conversation.

Children receive a diagnosis of autism when they meet the diagnostic criteria found in the *Diagnostic and Statistical Manual of Mental Disorders (DSM-IV-TR)* of the American Psychiatric Association. This book contains all the research-based information about mental disorders in both children and adults. The *DSM-IV-TR* criteria for autism are as follows:

A. Six or more items from (1), (2), and (3), with at least two from (1), and one each from (2) and (3):
   1. Qualitative impairment in social interaction, as manifested by at least two of the following:
      a. marked impairment in the use of multiple nonverbal behaviors such as eye-to-eye gaze, facial expression, body postures, and gestures to regulate social interaction

  b. failure to develop peer relationships appropriate to developmental level
  c. a lack of spontaneous seeking to share enjoyment, interests, or achievements with other people (e.g., by a lack of showing, bringing, or pointing out objects of interest)
  d. lack of social or emotional reciprocity
 2. Qualitative impairments in communication as manifested by at least one of the following:
  a. delay in, or total lack of, the development of spoken language (not accompanied by an attempt to compensate through alternative modes of communication such as a gesture or mime)
  b. in individuals with adequate speech, marked impairment in the ability to initiate or sustain a conversation with others
  c. stereotyped and repetitive use of language or idiosyncratic language
  d. lack of varied, spontaneous make-believe play or social imitative play appropriate to developmental level
 3. Restricted repetitive and stereotyped patterns of behavior, interests, and activities, as manifested by at least one of the following:
  a. encompassing preoccupation with one or more stereotyped and restricted patterns of interest that is abnormal either in intensity or focus
  b. apparently inflexible adherence to specific, nonfunctional routines or rituals
  c. stereotyped and repetitive motor manners (e.g., hand or finger flapping or twisting, or complex whole-body movements)
  d. persistent preoccupation with parts of objects
B. Delays or abnormal functioning in at least one of the following areas, with onset prior to age three years: (1) social interaction, (2) language as used in social communication, or (3) symbolic or imaginative play.[28]

As you can see, there's a lot of symptom manifestation in a child with autism. Some of these symptoms are subtle, others are more obvious. Most parents who have a child with autism report that they suspected something was wrong with their child long before the actual diagnosis was made.[29] Home videos of children's first birthdays reveal that children who are later diagnosed with autism exhibit significant differences in certain behaviors such as pointing, looking at others, and listening to other people talking.[30] Some of these behaviors were not noticed by parents at the time but were obvious when viewed later. This may explain why so many parents remain convinced that their child was developing perfectly normally until the child received vaccines. In addition, the age at which children should begin to become more socially interactive is around the same age as when the CDC recommends that children receive the first administration of most childhood vaccines. Since the coincidental timing of social development and vaccine administration is so close, it is understandable that parents might only notice their child's lack of social development at the same time their child receives the first course of vaccines.

Since the "onset" of autism appears, to parents, around the same time as the first vaccines, obviously the answer to the question "are vaccines and autism related?" should come from research studies that investigate that hypothesis. Such research has been done, in multiple countries, with multiple research groups, looking at many different variables. The overwhelming result of these studies is that vaccines are not related to autism.

It's estimated that approximately one child in 150 will be diagnosed with autism or an autism spectrum disorder at some point.[31] In comparison, one person in one hundred will be diagnosed with schizophrenia, a devastating mental illness, at some point. The anti-vaccine movement and the various autism advocacy groups cry about the modern epidemic of autism in our midst. With all the new vaccines that the CDC and pediatricians are recommending to parents, surely there's a connection, yes? No. And there are a number of explanations as to why the rates of autism are increasing.

It is true that in the 1990s, around the same time as the number of recommended childhood vaccines began to increase, the rates of autism began to increase as well. However, a review of the clinical literature indicates a couple of things. First, prior to 1994, the diagnostic criteria used were all over the place. Multiple diagnostic systems were used, which contaminates the data considerably, since diagnoses in one system might not necessarily line up with diagnoses arrived at using other systems. Since so many different "definitions" of autism were being used, any statements about diagnostic rates naturally depended on the system being used. Diagnoses using one set of criteria can't be combined with diagnoses using another set of criteria in any meaningful way.

Second, in 1994, the *DSM-IV* was published (the fourth edition of the diagnostic and statistical manual of the American Psychiatric Association, mentioned previously). This updated edition of the *DSM* included the aforementioned criteria, which were considerably more loosely defined than the original autism diagnostic criteria. The 1980 diagnostic criteria were much more rigid and demanded much more dysfunction. In addition, 1994 was the first time that Asperger's syndrome was included in the general category of autism spectrum disorders. Including this looser definition of autism, and allowing other disorders to be counted in the rates, meant there was an explosion of "new" diagnoses being made.

Finally, as rates of autism have supposedly risen, rates of mental retardation and other childhood developmental disorders have fallen. In some studies, that change is almost symmetrical. This is called "diagnostic substitution." It means that children who in previous generations might have received a diagnosis of mental retardation or developmental language disorder are now being diagnosed with autism. This diagnostic substitution makes it appear that rates are rising, when in reality, children are just receiving more appropriate diagnoses.[32]

Parents of children with any illness feel helpless, sometimes hopeless, often overwhelmed. It is natural for parents to look for a reason why their child has a disease or a disorder. Parents ask, "What did I do wrong? Did I take a medication at the wrong time of my pregnancy? Did I feed my child the wrong foods?" Parenting is a process that is filled with opportunities to second-guess your decisions or find blame for a negative outcome. In situations involving a disorder that is still so misunderstood, and for which we still do not have any good answers, it is understandable that parents would want to latch onto any possible explanation. Andrew Wakefield continues to insist that his research found a link between the MMR vaccine and autism, in spite of the evidence to the contrary. The anti-vaccine movement is not above lying or misrepresenting the scientific data. Finally, most parents aren't adequately trained in identifying what types of information are valid and what are not. These three forces all align to continue the perpetuation of the disproven myth.

In the meantime, autism rates continue to increase, in part for the reasons stated in this chapter and also for reasons still being investigated. Hundreds of millions of research dollars, and years of research effort, have all been wasted investigating a link that does not exist. There is never going to be enough scientific evidence to convince the dedicated anti-vaccine movement, and some parents, that there is no link between vaccines and autism. This is unfortunate, because the results of this ongoing conviction are clear—vaccine rates are falling, and the incidence of childhood vaccine-preventable diseases is rising. As a result of this mistaken belief, children are now dying of measles and whooping cough.

· 9 ·

Mark and David Geier:
Other Autism Myths

$\mathcal{T}$hanks to Andrew Wakefield's 1998 study, the anti-vaccine movement continues to focus on vaccines as the source of many childhood disorders. This focus has resulted in a number of people of dubious qualifications and ethics claiming they can "cure" these disorders. Most of these claims have no basis in science. Most of them come from people with little to no background in research or medicine. When the claims do come from people with backgrounds in medicine, parents can be all too easily misled. This is a dangerous situation. It results in the death of children undergoing unproven treatments and also contributes to the ongoing fearmongering about vaccines.

This chapter will talk about some of those claims and the people making them.

MARK AND DAVID GEIER

Mark Geier is a medical doctor based in Maryland. He has made a number of unproven claims regarding the safety of vaccines and the relationship between vaccines and autism. He has long been a supporter of the hypothesis linking the two. Even after the massive amount of research indicating the contrary, he continues to insist that autism is actually a form of mercury poisoning.[1] The idea that autism is mercury poisoning was originally published in a journal called *Medical Hypotheses*.[2] At the time, *Medical Hypotheses* had no peer-review process by which scientists would judge the scientific validity of the proposed articles. The journal is infamous for publishing articles denying that HIV causes AIDS, among other inaccurate and pseudoscientific information.

105

Dr. Geier's research and medical practice partner is his son, David Geier. David Geier has a bachelor's degree in biology, with a minor in history. He has no advanced training in biology, genetics, medicine, vaccines, or childhood developmental disorders. He is, however, his father's research partner in a number of publications that continue to insist on a link between vaccines and autism. He is also the president of MedCon, a consulting firm that specializes in helping people sue pharmaceutical companies.[3]

Dr. Mark Geier claims his research continually finds proof of a link between vaccines and autism. His research is widely considered by other scientists to be methodologically invalid for a variety of reasons. The primary reason is that he and his son frequently make use of the data in the Vaccine Adverse Event Reporting System (VAERS) in order to support his claims.

VAERS: USEFUL FOR SOME SITUATIONS, NOT FOR OTHERS

VAERS is a database that is jointly maintained by the CDC and the Food and Drug Administration (FDA).[4] As we discussed in chapter 6, it is designed to allow doctors and parents to report any suspected reaction to a vaccine. It also allows anyone, for any reason, to access certain parts of the database for information. The VAERS is open source, meaning anyone, anywhere, for any reason, can submit any report he wishes.

The VAERS was designed to allow the CDC and the FDA to identify patterns in public reporting. If a particular year, region, or vaccine starts to be associated with an increase in reported negative reactions, the CDC can take a more detailed look at that pattern. For example, in 1999 the VAERS system started receiving reports about the newly developed rotavirus vaccine. Those reports indicated that more children were experiencing certain intestinal reactions than would be expected. Because of the CDC verification and analysis of those reports, the vaccine was pulled and replaced by a safer version.[5]

For these reasons, the VAERS is a very useful public health tool. Researchers don't have to spend a lot of time and money to contact parents, health care professionals, or the general public to gather information. They can use the database to check for patterns reported by others. But this strength is also a weakness. Anyone can report any kind of vaccine reaction at any time. There are few to no checks on the validity of these reports. Indeed, in one humorous example, Dr. James Laidler deliberately submitted a report of himself turning into the Incredible Hulk after receiving a vaccine.[6] He did this in order to demonstrate that the VAERS database, while serving a public health need, is also incredibly flawed. Because reports can be submitted for any suspected reaction, even an obviously unrelated one, it is dangerous for any researcher to rely on the raw data in this source.

The VAERS data is not validated by the CDC or the FDA unless in extreme circumstances (such as the Incredible Hulk example) or for research purposes. Therefore, most of the reports received are never verified for accuracy. People viewing the database don't know if the reports are of real vaccine reactions or of reactions assumed to be related to vaccines. Since there is no review process, it is possible that someone can report a vaccine reaction even if she or her child never received a vaccine at all.

The timing of adverse reactions is also never verified. If a child has a fever one week after receiving a vaccine, some parents might report that as a vaccine reaction, while others might not. If a child gets a runny nose one day after being vaccinated, is the runny nose related to the vaccine or to a cold the child is developing? Some vaccine adverse reaction reports involve supposed reactions that occur weeks or months after immunization. Others involve reactions that occurred immediately.

As the anti-vaccine movement often points out, mild reactions, such as swelling or soreness at the injection site, are almost certainly underreported. Many people would not see these as worth reporting. If you get the flu vaccine and your arm feels a little achy, it would not occur to you to report that as a vaccine reaction. Severe illnesses that occur very soon after a vaccine would almost certainly be reported as a vaccine reaction even if the illness has nothing to do with the vaccine. Some parents who are already convinced that vaccines are dangerous would be significantly more likely to report anything out of the ordinary. Other parents might report only something frighteningly unusual, such as seizures in an otherwise healthy child.

In fact, many anti-vaccine advocates have engaged in campaigns designed to contaminate the database. They encourage parents of children with autism or other childhood disorders to report the disorder as a vaccine adverse reaction.[7] They do this regardless of whether the scientific research indicates the disorder is related to vaccines at all.

Analysis of the VAERS content indicates that reports to the database rise during certain times. Those times are related to vaccine-related lawsuits. When litigation about vaccines is occurring, litigation-related reports of adverse effects increase significantly.[8] In fact, it appears that some of those reports come directly from personal-injury lawyers as a deliberate attempt to contaminate the VAERS database.[9]

Finally, the VAERS reports by definition can be correlational only. A correlation is a relationship between two things. In this case, people assume there is a relationship between vaccines and adverse reactions. However, correlations don't tell you anything about cause and effect. They only tell you if two variables have a relationship. You cannot assume that one variable causes the other to happen. If researchers are going to find out if vaccines cause certain adverse effects, they need to use data that has many more controls than the VAERS database. The CDC even warns against using the VAERS information in such a manner.[10]

A better way of thinking about the VAERS is to consider it a system by which people can report medical conditions that occur after someone receives a vaccine. Since a broken leg cannot be caused by a vaccine, such a report would obviously not be considered a vaccine reaction. But what about a cold? The sniffles? A temper tantrum? A seizure three weeks after the DTaP vaccine? Whether or not these are adverse effects of the vaccines must be determined by the CDC and other researchers. Simply using the database to claim that all reported conditions are the result of vaccines is an inappropriate use of the data.

THE GEIERS AND THE VAERS

However, in many of their publications, the Geiers do exactly that. They frequently delve into the VAERS data without any sort of validation process whatsoever. They assume that every report of a vaccine-related adverse effect is valid and that each effect is directly caused by the vaccine in question. Since the VAERS database has been contaminated by false reports of vaccines causing autism, the Geiers' research naturally shows such a link.[11,12,13,14,15,16,17] But the data is invalid for this use. Garbage in, garbage out, as computer programmers always say.

In addition to perpetuating the myth that vaccines cause autism, the Geiers have developed a couple of controversial and dangerous treatments for children with autism.

The first involves a process called chelation. Chelation removes heavy metals such as lead or arsenic from the body. The process is used when someone has been exposed to dangerous levels of those metals. Such exposure is typically associated with industrial accidents or exposure over long periods of time, such as in a job working with hazardous materials. In chelation, chemicals are administered to the affected individual. These chemicals latch onto the heavy metals in the body, neutralize them, and help the body pass them through urine or fecal matter. Chelation is a relatively severe treatment reserved for critical conditions, and it has the potential for causing dangerous side effects and even death.[18,19]

The Geiers have proposed that chelation can help children with autism by removing excess mercury in their bodies. Again, the theory that autism is mercury poisoning has no scientific validity. That hasn't stopped the Geiers from convincing desperate parents to try this dangerous procedure. They claim the urine tests they administer to patients reveal high levels of heavy metals. In fact, they administer chelating agents prior to urine testing, creating an unnatural release of metals already in the body. This unnatural release makes the urine artificially high in metals, and the Geiers use these levels to "prove" that children with autism have heavy metal poisoning.[20] They then convince parents to spend thousands of dollars on supplements and treatments designed to leach those heavy metals from their children's bodies. Needless to say, such treatments have absolutely no scientific validity.[21,22] At least one child with autism has already died from chelation therapy.[23]

TESTOSTERONE: THE GEIERS' HOLY GRAIL

Of course, chelation doesn't work on children with developmental disorders. Heavy metal poisoning is associated with brain damage but not with autism. There is no evidence that autism is related to heavy metal poisoning or mercury poisoning. Vaccines are not a source of mercury poisoning.

In spite of the fact that from a biological standpoint, chelation therapy cannot have any therapeutic effects on autism, the Geiers claimed the therapy was successful in treating some children with autism. However, when chelation therapy did not cure some of their patients, the Geiers developed a theory related to testosterone in the human body. According to this theory, excess testosterone increases the toxicity of mercury.[24] The Geiers claim that it does so by binding to the mercury and preventing it from being processed out of the body naturally. Therefore, children with autism were suffering both from mercury poisoning *and* from excess testosterone. There is no scientific evidence to support this theory.

It is true that autism affects boys more often than girls. There are numerous studies addressing this gender inequality. Some of the research indicates that genetic abnormalities on the X chromosome might be involved. Any time a genetic mutation or abnormality involves the X chromosome, boys are significantly more likely to be affected than girls. Girls have two X chromosomes, so if something is wrong with one of their X chromosomes, the likelihood is that the other one will be normal. The normal chromosome can then compensate for the non-normal one. However, boys have only one

X chromosome. Therefore, if that chromosome is abnormal, the Y chromosome cannot compensate for the abnormality. That's why hemophilia, fragile X, and many other X-linked chromosomal abnormalities are going to affect more boys than girls.

It's normal to wonder if testosterone, as well as X-linked abnormalities, is part of the difference between male and female autism rates. After all, men have more testosterone than women, so looking at differences in the effects of testosterone on differences in autism rates is a natural research direction. Some research has shown that in animals, testosterone may increase the damaging effects of mercury. However, some research has shown the opposite—that testosterone protects against mercury damage. Therefore, the relationship between mercury poisoning and testosterone is still unclear.[25] Of course, the relationship between mercury poisoning and testosterone is irrelevant to the issue of autism, since autism is not caused by mercury poisoning.

The lack of scientific evidence regarding the effect of testosterone on mercury poisoning (which is not a cause of autism) has not stopped the Geiers from developing yet another unproven and dangerous treatment.

PRECOCIOUS PUBERTY AND LUPRON: CASTRATING LITTLE BOYS

The Geiers, based on the unpublished and unproven theory that testosterone increases the effects of mercury in the body, developed a protocol for treating boys with autism. They began to determine that children with autism actually have a condition known as precocious puberty. Precocious puberty is a condition in which the secondary sex characteristics (for example, pubic hair for both genders, breasts for girls, facial hair and voice deepening for boys) appear earlier than normal. Normal puberty occurs around nine to fourteen years of age for girls and around twelve to sixteen years of age for boys, although that varies based on ethnicity. In precocious puberty, the secondary sex characteristics appear prior to the age of eight for girls and nine for boys. This condition is relatively uncommon and is seen significantly more often in girls than boys.[26]

Generally, the treatment for precocious puberty is to address the underlying cause, if one can be identified. For example, if the changes are due to a tumor, the tumor is removed. However, in most cases of precocious puberty, there is no underlying cause. In those cases, the children are treated with medication to delay the onset of puberty.[27]

The Geiers diagnosed a significant percentage of the children with autism that they have seen in their medical offices with precocious puberty.[28] Claiming the increased testosterone associated with precocious puberty is interacting with the mercury poisoning from the vaccines, they then set about reducing the amount of testosterone in the children's bodies. They did this using a medicine called Lupron.[29]

Lupron is a drug that reduces the production of estradiol and testosterone in the body. It is used for treating endometriosis and uterine fibroids in women as well as certain cancers that respond to hormone decreases. It has also been used in cases involving sex offenses. Males who have committed sexual assaults have occasionally been given the opportunity to undergo what is known as chemical castration. This involves giving them enough Lupron to theoretically decrease their testosterone levels to the point where they will no longer experience sexual desire. The use of Lupron as a chemical castrating agent is controversial in the criminal justice system.

Apparently, the use of Lupron as a treatment for vaccine-related autism is not, as the Geiers developed, patented, and marketed the treatment protocol to hundreds of parents over the years.[30] The developer of Lupron, Abbott Laboratories, once applied for a treatment protocol patent with the Geiers but is no longer involved with that partnership, stating there is no scientific evidence to support the venture.

THE GEIERS: BUSINESS AND LEGAL MISCONDUCT

Dr. Mark Geier is the current president of Genetic Centers of America. He is one of the most widely used expert witnesses for the prosecution in vaccine-related litigation. He is frequently the only expert witness in these cases, in which people sue vaccine manufacturers for supposed vaccine-related adverse effects. He testifies against vaccine manufacturers, using his scientifically invalid research as his "proof" that vaccines are dangerous. He then requests to be compensated for his time and expertise. These requests often include fees that are not allowed in the courts.

Dr. Geier has been declared untrustworthy and unreliable as an expert witness by a number of different judges. His testimony has been labeled fraudulent, inaccurate, and unsupported. In fact, he has been warned by several judges to cease misrepresenting his background, training, and expertise. He claims to have credentials he does not possess, and he has been sanctioned for doing so.

In 2010, his behavior was determined to be so egregious that his medical license was suspended in Maryland. That suspension was followed by suspensions of his medical license in Washington, Virginia, and California. He still holds a current medical license in several states.

David Geier, Dr. Geier's son, is the president of MedCon. MedCon advertises itself as a consulting group that assists people in suing vaccine manufacturers. The address of MedCon is the same address as Mark Geier's private residence. David Geier frequently submits bills to vaccine courts to be compensated for his expertise, in spite of the fact that he possesses no advanced degrees in biology, genetics, or the law. He claims to have received some advanced training in the areas of vaccines and immunology, among others. The bills submitted by David Geier and his father have been determined to be excessive and for unnecessary and unrelated expenses.

In 2009, David Geier was named to the Maryland Commission on Autism, regardless of his lack of credentials. After his father's medical license was suspended in 2010, the Maryland autism board removed David Geier from its membership. When asked why an obviously unqualified person with such a clear conflict of interest had been able to gain an appointment to the board, the board spokesperson stated that at the time of his appointment, it was felt that having "different perspectives" was beneficial to the board's mission.[31]

During the same year, the State of Maryland charged David Geier with practicing medicine without a license.[32] David Geier is listed as the executive director of ASD Centers, LLC, which is a center that describes itself on its home page as "physician-owned and operated." It exists to help parents of autistic children find treatments for their children's disorder. In a formal document from the State of Maryland, David Geier was accused of seeing four different children at the ASD in Maryland and performing medical examinations on all four children. The parents of the four children stated in the complaint that they were under the impression David Geier was a physician. He ordered a number of unnecessary tests in these cases, as well as charged for office visits that did not take place.[33]

SCIENTIFIC MISCONDUCT

All research performed on human or animal subjects must undergo review by an institutional review board (IRB). The IRB reviews any proposed research to ensure that animal or human subjects are being treated ethically. The IRB also determines whether or not the research is necessary and would contribute to the scientific body of knowledge. IRBs in the United States are sanctioned by the FDA and the Department of Health and Human Services. These sanctions ensure that the IRBs so recognized are valid and legitimate scientific bodies.[34]

The IRB for Dr. Mark Geier's research in the use of Lupron for treating autism is the Institute for Chronic Illness (ICI). The ICI is a nonprofit corporation in Silver Springs, Maryland, with the same address as the home address of Mark Geier. The IRB for ICI consists of Mark Geier, his wife Anne, his son David Geier, his ASD Centers partner, and the parents of several of his patients. None of these listed members possess the advanced training or scientific credentials expected of an independent and valid IRB. It is also highly unusual for scientific research to be conducted, at least on paper, out of one's private residence.[35]

Mark and David Geier are two of the major perpetrators of inaccurate and disproven information regarding the safety and efficacy of vaccines. First, they continue to spread the myth that vaccines are related to autism, in spite of the massive amounts of scientific evidence to the contrary. The only evidence they cite is their own research, which uses the VAERS database in incorrect and invalid ways. They then maintain that autism is a form of mercury poisoning, a claim not supported by scientific information. They assert that a dangerous treatment, chelation therapy, will remove that poisoning. When that doesn't work, they diagnose the child with precocious puberty and use a chemical castration drug to treat the condition.

None of these claims are accurate. None are backed up by research. All of them are dangerous to the children involved.

· *10* ·

ADHD, Allergies, and All the Rest: Other Vaccine Myths

$\mathcal{A}$nti-vaccine websites warn parents that vaccines cause problems in addition to autism. They blame vaccines for a whole host of illnesses and conditions. They call these conditions vaccine injuries.

Let's talk about those myths and the science that disproves them.

ADHD: NOT JUST NORMAL KID BEHAVIOR

One of the most controversial children's diagnoses is attention deficit disorder. It is referred to in the *DSM-IV* as Attention Deficit Hyperactivity Disorder (ADHD), with two subtypes. One of the subtypes is Predominantly Inattentive (ADHD-PI), and the other subtype is Predominantly Hyperactive (ADHD-PH). So a child could be diagnosed with ADHD but not be hyperactive. A child could also have both hyperactive and inattentive symptoms. It's complicated, but the guiding principle in both subtypes is that the child has trouble paying attention.

That trouble can take two different forms. The stereotype of the child with ADHD-PI is that the child can't focus. Children are seen jumping from one topic to another or are often accused of daydreaming. They seem to drift off mentally. However, it is also possible that the child can be intensely focused on a task to the exclusion of everything else. The child with ADHD-PI might spend hours focused on a single book yet not be able to pay attention to a conversation. This problem with attention is to a level that is dysfunctional—it interferes with the child's ability to function as expected.

When most people think of ADHD, they think of a hyperactive child. This is the child who runs around all the time. A child who fidgets constantly. Who can't stay seated in a chair for more than thirty seconds. Who interrupts conversations or blurts out answers in school. A child who seems wired on energy all the time. This level of energy is not normal child energy but activity and energy that are dysfunctional. It interferes with the child's ability to participate appropriately in life. This is the primarily hyperactive subtype.

The *DSM-IV* diagnostic criteria for both subtypes are pretty extensive. It's important to keep that in mind. Many people claim that ADHD doesn't exist. They state that normal children exhibiting normal child behavior are being labeled and medicated. They point to the rising rates of diagnosis as proof that doctors and teachers are just interested in drugging children.

The key criterion, one that many people don't know, is that the behaviors have to be present in two or more environments. Many people claim that children who are bored in school get "labeled" with ADHD. However, a child who exhibits the symptoms only at school does not qualify for the diagnosis. The child has to exhibit these dysfunctional symptoms at school and in at least one more setting. That setting can be home, or religious settings, or community activities. But exhibiting those behaviors in one setting is not enough for the child to receive a diagnosis of ADHD of either subtype.

The debate regarding ADHD is too long, too large, and too complicated to adequately discuss in one chapter. However, scientists are doing research into the causes of the disorder in order to develop better treatments and possibly identify a way to intervene. Reducing any contributing factors would go a long way to figuring out whether the disorder is "real" or not.

Therefore, of course, scientists are looking at lots of different hypotheses. Vaccines are a part of that research.

VACCINES AND ADHD: WHAT THE SCIENCE SHOWS

Obviously, some researchers who investigated possible links between vaccines and autism also looked at possible links between vaccines and other disorders. Very early and superficial research appeared to find a link between vaccines and lots of developmental disorders.[1] That early research contained some methodological issues, as is typical for newer research in a field. It also operated under the old assumption that ethylmercury and methylmercury had the same effects in the body. Finally, the findings in the research were complicated by variables that weren't separated out (called confounding variables). Researchers then followed up with this early research by using more valid models.

Researchers in the United Kingdom looked at all children born between 1988 and 1997 who were followed by the health care system for at least two years. They ended up with a very large subject pool of 107,152 children. Since this was another study looking at thimerosal, they calculated the amount of thimerosal the children had received. At the time, the DTP and DT vaccines were the only childhood vaccines in the United Kingdom that contained thimerosal. The researchers looked at the levels of thimerosal and any diagnoses the children received. They eliminated children with confounding diagnoses such as Down syndrome, cerebral palsy, and head injuries. They found no relationship between vaccines received, levels of thimerosal, and any diagnosis of attention deficit disorders.[2]

Another study from Britain was published at the same time as this one. Instead of looking back at medical records, the researchers in the second group followed a group of children from birth. The first type of study is called retrospective, while the second type of study is called prospective. When used together, these two types of studies can provide a clearer picture of the issue. The researchers in the second group followed 12,956 children born between April 1, 1991, and December 31, 1992. They assessed a number of behavioral and developmental outcomes at 6, 18, 30, 47, 81, and 91 months of age. They also calculated the amount of thimerosal exposure over the course of those subjects' vaccine records. They, too, found no link between the amount of thimerosal exposure and any developmental disorders, including ADHD.[3]

In 2007, an American research group looked at 1,107 children between the ages of seven and ten. They assessed the children with a wide variety of tests for various developmental milestones, including IQ, language development, and attention. They then correlated those test results with the amount of thimerosal the children had received over the course of their childhood vaccine schedules. Again, they found no link between any developmental disorders and thimerosal.[4]

ADHD: IF NOT VACCINES, THEN WHAT?

Again, as with autism, scientists are not sure. The research into contributing factors for ADHD is looking at several possibilities. There is evidence of a genetic component, as the disorder runs in families.[5] Parents with certain disorders are more likely to have children with ADHD and other childhood disruptive disorders.[6] Siblings are also likely to share disorders.[7] Research indicates that multiple genes are involved.[8]

Brain structure and brain function seem to be different in children with ADHD. Some researchers found differences in levels of neurotransmitters, the chemicals used by the brain cells to communicate with each other.[9] Other scientists have found functional differences in many different brain areas.[10,11,12] Some studies found differences in brain structures or brain volume.[13,14] In some cases, the brains of children with ADHD seem to develop slower than the brains of children without the disorder.[15]

Environmental factors seem to play a part as well. Some research has found that early TV exposure is associated with attention problems,[16] but that research is inconsistent. Exposure to pesticides appears to increase the risk of ADHD.[17,18] Other risk factors include low birth weight, exposure to alcohol or cigarette smoke in utero, or complications in childbirth.[12]

The exact cause of ADHD is still unknown at this time. The research indicates that the disorder is probably a result of interactions between genetic, biological, and environmental factors. However, vaccines have been ruled out as a contributing factor.

It is interesting that the amount of scientific research into a link between vaccines and ADHD is not as extensive as the research about autism. There are a couple of probable explanations for that difference. First, many people still insist that ADHD is not a "real" disorder. Others believe that while it may be a real disorder, it's overdiagnosed (but those people never say how often they think it *should* be diagnosed). Still others think it's a result of bad or lazy parenting. The lack of wide acceptance of the validity of the disorder may be inhibiting research.

The second possible explanation is that overall, autism has a tendency to be more devastating to a child's ability to function. Most children with ADHD can still function at some level, even if that functioning is significantly affected. However, in the cases of severe autism, the child's functioning is significantly more limited. Since research dollars are scarce, researchers may feel the more problematic disorder should be the highest priority.

ALLERGIES

Allergies occur when the body's immune system overreacts to the presence of a substance. That substance can be ingested, such as food; inhaled, such as pollen; or touched, such as poison ivy. Substances that trigger allergies are called allergens. Some allergies are mild, while others can be life-threatening.

Approximately 20 percent of the American population suffers from some form of allergies, including asthma.[19]

The unpredictable nature of allergies makes them a concern for many parents. Feeding on that understandable concern, the anti-vaccine movement claims that vaccines increase the likelihood of childhood allergies. The research does not support that claim.

In 1998, researchers published a study of 669 children. The children were randomly divided into four groups. The first three groups each received a different type of pertussis vaccine, and the last group received a vaccine that did not contain any active ingredient (a placebo). The random assignment of subjects into various groups is a hallmark of good research. Random assignment means that each child had an equal chance of being in each group. It allows scientists to spread any individual differences among the groups. The results from this design can then be said to be free of chance differences.

The scientists assessed the children with skin prick tests for allergies at seven months and two and a half years of age. There was no difference in allergies between any of the four groups.[20] In 2003, those same researchers reassessed those same children at age seven and found no differences in allergies between three of the four groups. The fourth group showed a slight increase in allergies, but those children had received an experimental vaccine that was no longer used.[21]

A larger study, with more subjects, was published in 2004. It looked at data from 1988 through 1999 from a large medical database in England. Some of the children had received the measles, mumps, and rubella (MMR) vaccine only. Other children had received the diphtheria, polio, pertussis, and tetanus (DPPT) vaccine, and still others had received both vaccines. Researchers compared rates of allergies between all three groups and found no differences.[22]

Again, multiple studies investigated any possible links between vaccines and allergies. Those studies continually find no link. This is true for multiple types of vaccines.[23,24,25,26] The research has been done in multiple countries.[27,28,29,30] Once again, the overwhelming scientific consensus is that there is no link between vaccines and allergies.[31]

ASTHMA

Asthma occurs when the airways constrict or become blocked. This causes breathing difficulties that can result in gasping, wheezing, or choking. If asthma is triggered by an allergen such as pollen, it is called allergic, or extrinsic, asthma. If asthma is triggered by something else, such as stress, cold air, or exercise, it is called nonallergic, or intrinsic, asthma.

In most of the allergy studies already discussed, researchers looked at extrinsic asthma as well as the other allergies. Therefore, the scientific data from those studies would apply to this type of allergy. In addition, researchers often investigate asthma by itself instead of including it in general allergy research. As with autism, ADHD, and allergies, the research results are clear.

Researchers followed 167,240 children from the years 1991 to 1997. These children were enrolled as patients with several large HMOs. The researchers followed them all for a minimum of eighteen months of age and a maximum of six years of age. They correlated any diagnoses of asthma with five different vaccines: the MMR vaccine, the oral polio vaccine (OPV), the DTP vaccine, the Hib vaccine, and the hepatitis B vaccine. Researchers found no link between any of these five different vaccines and the development of asthma.[32]

Perhaps the best evidence that vaccines have no relationship to asthma comes from the International Study of Asthma and Allergies in Childhood (ISAAC). ISAAC is a collaborative study involving, as of 2011, almost two million children from 105 countries. The study was originally divided into three phases, but a fourth phase has been added since the onset of the study. Phase one involved gathering data from 155 locations in 56 countries. There were 721,601 children studied. Data was gathered regarding rates of asthma and allergies in six- and seven-year-olds and in thirteen- and fourteen-year olds. That data was correlated with vaccination histories. Phase one of ISAAC found no relationship between the DTP, tuberculosis, or measles vaccines.[33]

The causes of asthma, like the causes of other allergies, are still under investigation. Asthma appears to be related to complex genetic factors.[34] Air pollution, both indoor and outdoor, has been identified as at least exacerbating asthma, if not causing it.[35,36] Ozone concentrations[37] and other atmospheric contributing factors have been identified. One theory is that children are being raised in households that are too clean. The increased use of antibacterial products or antibiotics leads children to have fewer low-level infections during childhood, which contributes to an immune system that overreacts by manifesting asthma.[38] Scientists are attempting to determine whether any or all of these factors cause asthma, exacerbate asthma, or do both.

Asthma, like allergies and ADHD, is a complex disorder with many factors. Vaccines have been ruled out as one of those factors.

DIABETES

The anti-vaccine movement claims that vaccines contribute to the development of diabetes. Science, once again, has investigated this claim and found no support.

Diabetes is a metabolic disorder. People with diabetes do not release enough insulin from the pancreas to adequately process their food into glucose. Glucose is the fuel that our cells use to function. Some people do not produce any insulin at all (type I diabetes), while others do not produce enough insulin (type II). There is also a type of diabetes that occurs in pregnant women (gestational diabetes).

People with diabetes can experience mild symptoms that do not significantly interfere with their lives. On the other hand, people with diabetes can experience life-threatening symptoms, such as kidney failure or gangrene in the extremities due to death of the tissues. Some people with diabetes can control their condition with diet, exercise, and other modifications of their lifestyles. Others require lifelong medication in order to survive.

The United States has experienced a significant increase in the rates of diabetes over the past several decades.[39] Because that increase is occurring at the same time as available immunizations increase, it's natural that people will link the two. Let's look at the research.

Some preliminary studies in fact appeared to find a link between vaccines and the development of type I diabetes.[40] However, there were methodological flaws in these early studies. The researchers in the original studies, D. C. Classen and J. B. Classen, are well known in the anti-vaccine movement. They have filed patents regarding the timing of immunizations based on their research. They claim that early (within one month of birth) immunization prevents diabetes, but later immunizations cause diabetes.[41] Follow-up research from multiple countries was not able to locate the claimed relationship between vaccines and diabetes.[42,43,44,45]

As with the other disorders discussed in this chapter, the causes of diabetes are complex. Multiple genetic factors have been studied and identified for both type I and type II diabetes.[46,47] Physical risk factors such as obesity and a lack of exercise have also been identified.[48,49] Diabetes, especially type 2, seems to be more prevalent in certain ethnic groups.[50] Environmental risk factors for type 1 diabetes include increased maternal age and in-utero infections.[51]

Vaccines are not a contributing factor to diabetes.

OBESITY: AN INCREASING ISSUE, IN EVERY SENSE

All you have to do is turn on the television or pick up a newspaper to know that obesity is a public health epidemic. This isn't true just for the United States—it's also true for most of the developed world.[52] The primary reasons for the increase in size are pretty well known to public health professionals. People in developed countries have more access to more calorie-dense food now than in past generations. At the same time, we are moving less. We walk, bike, hike, run, dance, and play sports less than in past generations. This imbalance between energy consumed (in food) and energy expended (through activity) creates obesity.[53]

Certainly, there are some medical disorders that cause obesity even when the person's intake of food and output of energy is balanced. Some genetic and metabolic disorders contribute to the development of obesity.[54] These disorders are estimated to cause only about 1 percent of obesity.[55]

Naturally, people want to find out if there are other factors contributing to the obesity epidemic. Some scientists have identified certain viruses that cause obesity in humans and animals.[56,57] None of those viruses are found in childhood or adult vaccines. The anti-vaccine movement claims that ingredients in vaccines (such as sucrose) cause childhood obesity. There is no scientific evidence for this statement.

WHY THE MYTHS?

If there's no scientifically proven link between vaccines and any of these disorders, then why does a belief in these links still exist? For the same reasons the myth of a link between vaccines and autism exists. People want answers. Parents want an explanation for their child's medical problems. Understandably, parents are not satisfied with a "we're not sure" response from medical personal. This kind of answer leaves a hole in the parents' conception of the world.

It's easy for people to fill that hole with unproven hysteria. People are attracted to information that appears, on the surface, to provide an explanation. Most of the anti-vaccine movement's claims sound plausible at first glance. Most parents aren't science experts or doctors. The scientific claims put forth regarding the links between vaccines and these disorders are sometimes difficult to assess without training in biology or scientific methodology. So, frightened and confused parents are vulnerable to being misled.

Add to that the belief that modern medicine should know by now what causes these disorders. Haven't we been studying them for decades? We have, but the complexity of these disorders makes it difficult for scientists to pick out a single cause for any of them. The truth of the matter is that all these disorders are created by a combination of genetic and environmental factors. But vaccines are not one of those environmental factors that contribute to ADHD, allergies, asthma, diabetes, or obesity.

· // ·

The Good, the Bad, and the Ugly:
A Guide to the Online World

*A*ccess to good information is vital. Without it we are all lost. The topic of vaccines is no different. Basic information about vaccination can be gleaned from any book including this one. However, the field of vaccination science is not static. New vaccines are constantly in development. Many vaccine makers reformulate old vaccines in an effort to help make them safer. From yearly flu shots to changing guidelines about the need for boosters or changing state mandates, access to reliable and updated information on vaccines is critical to anyone interested in the subject.

One of the first places many people turn to for information about vaccines is the Internet. Most Americans have Internet access at home, work, or both. Many others can easily gain access via the local public library or community center. As a result, the Internet serves as one of the most important areas of dissemination about vaccines.

While the Internet is an extremely useful tool, it has several drawbacks that users must always be mindful of when reading any site. It's important to keep in mind how websites are constructed, as well as the kind of information that may be found on those websites, before you begin. Not all information sources are created equal. Some contain information that is not only actively misleading but might also be factually untrue. Learning to spot the problems with any given site and find sites that offer good information allows you to stay on top of the latest developments in this field. This knowledge allows parents to become empowered, form their own effective understanding of any changes in vaccine scheduling, and ask informed questions of local health authorities and their own pediatricians. You don't even need specific knowledge of biology or chemistry to do so. A little common sense and some understanding of how to look closely at a website will suffice.

HOW TO SET UP A WEBSITE IN FIVE EASY STEPS

One of the great glories of the Internet is that people from all over the world can connect with each other. Someone from Scotland can speak directly to someone in the Seychelles. Those two can build a website to connect with even more people, and this exponential connection can occur quickly and easily. However, this very benefit comes with a price. The ease of Internet communication makes bad information that much more difficult to track down and correct, let alone eradicate. Conspiracy theories that might have circulated just around the block for a few days before the Internet can now circulate around an entire globe in a day or less. While you might shrug if your mother-in-law Marilyn sends out yet another deceptive e-mail filled with silly allegations about the evils of spaying a pet or how a specific political candidate is allegedly forging his birth certificate, you might be more inclined to take her seriously if she sends you a link to what appears to be a well-crafted website.

Any website can appear quite authoritative at first glance. A site filled with well-chosen imagery and that links to what appear to be accurate scientific studies and moving testimonials can fool even informed observers.

A website is not that difficult to set up. Anyone can create a website with a few simple steps. All you really need is a reliable outside host with enough computing power, a blog, access to a database that allows you to use pictures for free, and a basic command of your native language. The hosting service ensures that your site stays up. Any blog can be customized to suit your needs. You can pick and choose from free templates or buy specialized templates from outside sources that specialize in Web design. Website owners can essentially do what they want once the site is set up. A site owner can add daily updates, link to other websites, buy pictures to use, and sell products. The owner can allow users to comment, can delete comments deemed offensive, and can allow other people to link to the site without penalty.

Perhaps even more important, a website that looks pleasing to most people and seems credible on reasonable first examination can be set up at minimal cost and maintained indefinitely for less than the price of the average monthly phone bill. Allowing advertising from local authorities or Google AdWords and/or selling products can easily offset any minor costs the owner might otherwise incur. Clearly, spreading good or bad information via a personal website is quite simple and inexpensive to do.

The Internet has very few police or filters. Aside from a few taboo subjects such as illicit drug use and child pornography, search engines allow people to create sites about nearly any subject they want. Website owners are in charge of their sites and do not answer to anyone at Google or any outside authority. More important, search engines allow users to find data from such sites. Google, Bing, and Yahoo! are not checking to see if the data you find is accurate. The search engine does not care.

This applies to medical data as well. With the right marketing and reasonably well-written articles, even a site alleging that a cure for cancer is secretly being kept in a vault on Mars can easily get ranked by any search engine. Most users will click on the first three or four results they see, at least initially, on the presumption that Google or Yahoo! knows what they need.

The only possible penalty for websites that search engines perceive as bad is that such websites may drop in the search rankings. For example, if Google determines a site does not fit a searcher's needs, contains poorly written information, or plagiarizes information from somewhere else, Google officials may decide to drop the site from the top ten results, relegate it ten pages away, or refuse to rank it altogether. Or the site may remain in the search results with no indication of the problematic content.

HOW TO DO A BASIC SEARCH FOR ANSWERS TO QUESTIONS ABOUT VACCINES

Searching the Web for information is both a science and an art form. Ideally you want your specific questions answered. You also want places to turn to for additional information related to your original query.

Google is the most widely used search engine, but it is not the only search engine you can use. Many medical professionals work with search engines that focus on medical information. They are designed to filter out information from websites judged to lack proper scientific credentials. Using such tools allows you to search for information from sources such as scientific journals available to the public online and popular websites with sources that have been fact-checked such as CNN. Google also has a feature called Google Scholar, which limits Google searches to only scientific journal articles and other valid sources.

Medical search engines include pogofrog.com, omnimedicalsearch.com, webmd.com, healthfinder.gov, and pubmed.gov. PogoFrog is designed primarily for use by medical professionals but offers many articles of interest to the layman as well. Healthfinder is a service maintained by the U.S. Department of Health and Human Services. The site gathers information from over 1,600 sources on all sorts of health topics, including vaccines. PubMed lets users directly search through millions of medical journal articles. Some are available only as abstracts unless you have a paid subscription. Many, if not most, articles can be viewed in their entirety for free.

Any search engine search will bring up a list of dozens of websites you can check out directly. A website is not a guarantee of anything at all. Websites can be used for all sorts of purposes including selling products and even allowing people to gather together and spread disinformation or insult people based on their race or sex. Be very cautious when reading any information about vaccines on websites found through a general search engine.

Ideally, the best search strategy is to use multiple specialized search engines. A Google search on vaccines will generate very different results from a Google Scholar search on vaccines. The first will pull results from all over the Internet, including unsubstantiated personal websites. The second will pull only results from academically and scientifically valid sources. When you are interested in doing an Internet search on medical information, you will get the best results by using more than one of the aforementioned specialized search engines.

Just as not all websites are created equal, not all medical journals are created equal. Some journals are not peer reviewed and are open to submissions from nearly anyone, just as some magazines and blogs allow nearly anyone to comment or submit. This may sound surprising to someone without medical or scientific training, but it's true.

Many websites with an anti-vaccine slant will appear on the surface to contain lots of references to medical information from what looks like legitimate sources. Often, the number of these references is overwhelming to the casual Web surfer, tending to decrease the likelihood that the reader will actually read them all. This technique has been dubbed "Gish Gallop." Duane Gish is a biochemist who argues against the scientific fact of biological evolution. Gish is known for hauling out massive amounts of information during a debate that initially appears legitimate but does not hold up to further scrutiny when examined more closely. Many anti-vaccine websites employ a similar method. They are often filled with dozens of references to what appear to be scientifically valid journals and articles. However, closer examination often reveals the very opposite.

FOUR HALLMARKS OF A GOOD MEDICAL WEBSITE

All the previously mentioned factors apply to websites related to vaccines or any other medical issue. No specific authority has been set up to look closely at any website offering information about vaccines. No one will tell you if the information presented is written by someone with an advanced degree in biology or someone with a product to sell.

You have to figure this out yourself. Fortunately, this is fairly easy. A reliable website should follow several basic guidelines when you read it.

The first important principle is transparency. It should be obvious exactly who is presenting the information. If you go to the World Health Organization's website, you know immediately that you are there. A site should tell you who runs it. If you don't see this information, you may have to dig around for it by looking at sections such as the "about us" link or contact information.

Another important indication of a reliable website is the way the information is presented. Read all headlines on the home page. A headline describing scientific information should avoid bias and sensationalism and use accurate and accepted terminology. The headline or title "Copper Bracelets Cure Arthritis!" is to be viewed with suspicion, whereas the headline or title "Scientific data on the use of copper bracelets and the alleviation of arthritis symptoms" is impartial and reasonable.

Reliable medical websites avoid overt commercialization. Most websites allow advertising, and many allow links to products. Advertising is not all bad. Royalties from a good product can help a site remain in business. But the site should not be plastered with advertising underneath every single paragraph. A site dedicated to a medical condition should sell only products of scientifically proven value. Sites offering products that make outrageous claims such as a complete cure for all cancers should immediately raise red flags.

Funding sources should be obvious and easily identified. For example, the National Network for Immunization Information website states, "Neither NNii nor its sponsoring corporation, I4PH, accept any financial support from the pharmaceutical industry or the federal government."[1]

A trustworthy website should also link to good external sources of information. Some websites will direct you to other websites that are obviously filled with errors. A website should send you only to other equally valid sites. Look for links to information from the latest studies in respected medical journals.

THE GOOD . . .

While the Internet has some really bad information, it also offers even casual users a treasure trove of truly good information. You can access the good websites for answers to nearly any question at any hour of the day.

Here are some of our favorite websites about vaccines. So the next time your neighbor or your dimwitted sister-in-law or that long lost cousin you found on Facebook sends you a list of why vaccines are bad, you can do a quick search and refute their arguments. These sites are easy to navigate, written in layman's terms, and go into great detail about any remaining questions you might have about this subject. All the sites in question have information that has been vetted by medical authorities. Many have articles on vaccines that are updated on a weekly and even daily basis. Most also have sections geared toward parents and interested professionals who do not have a scientific background.

The American Academy of Pediatrics The American Academy of Pediatrics (AAP) represents over sixty thousand American pediatricians. The AAP's website provides users with instant access to reliable information about children's health. The site has a specific area devoted to vaccines. Parents can find up-to-date information about vaccination schedules, safety issues, and local community resources.

The Centers for Disease Control and Prevention The CDC has a huge online website devoted to vaccines. The CDC is a part of the U.S. Department of Health and Human Services and thus funded by the American government. The section of the website on vaccines offers a comprehensive examination of all aspects of vaccination. Parents can search through the database to find specific information about vaccines for their children from birth to adolescence. The CDC also maintains a hotline where you can speak to health professionals directly about this issue.

The Immunization Action Coalition The Immunization Action Coalition (IAC) is a nonprofit organization that lobbies to increase community vaccination rates. The IAC's website offers parents hundreds of pages of information about vaccine-preventable diseases. Under the section for parents, you'll find information about topics such as state vaccine mandates, tips for searching out old information records, and what to do if you are traveling to a foreign country with a baby or toddler. The website also includes quite graphic pictures that illustrate what someone with an advanced case of measles or tetanus looks like.

The National Network for Immunization Information The NNii has been set up to provide people with information about the latest developments in vaccines. The information on the site is aimed at both health professionals and parents. Parents can find very detailed information about vaccines in the vaccination schedule, including the name of the manufacturer, the year the vaccine was initially licensed, potential side effects, and the percentage of people who will be immune to the disease after being vaccinated.

Parents of Kids with Infectious Diseases Founded in 1996, Parents of Kids with Infectious Diseases (PKID) is an organization devoted to helping children with potentially contagious diseases and their caregivers. The organization aims to dispel the many myths surrounding children living with diseases such as AIDS and hepatitis. Its website offers support and information about vaccine-preventable diseases for parents who have children who may have been born too early to get vaccinated or who did not have access to vaccination in their home countries. The information provided also comes from medical professionals. Parents can submit questions about vaccine-preventable diseases to health professionals via e-mail directly from the website.

The Vaccine Education Center at the Children's Hospital of Philadelphia The Vaccine Education Center is a nonprofit organization at the Children's Hospital of Philadelphia. The Children's Hospital of Philadelphia was the nation's first pediatric hospital and has continued to provide quality care for children ever since. The Vaccine Education Center aims to help parents separate myth from facts on vaccines. Visitors to the hospital's website can access a tremendous amount of information about immunizations including webinars, free videos, and a very detailed look at each individual vaccine. The site is updated frequently so you can always find the latest information about new vaccines and answers to any ongoing concerns you may have.

The Vaccine Resource Library The Vaccine Resource Library is funded by PATH, or the Program for Appropriate Technology in Health. PATH is a nonprofit organization that aims to work with governments around the world to improve their health care systems and help people protect themselves against illness. The Vaccine Resource Library contains thousands of links to useful articles on vaccines from health professionals and science writers around the world. Parents in search of well-written and informative data can easily find it here.

AND THE BAD

In our opinion, some websites that focus on vaccines are, quite honestly, simply awful. Such websites contain not only misleading information but also outright lies. We feel they deserve to be called out. So we're doing just that. On these sites you'll find deceptive statistics, exaggerated claims, and outright conspiracy theories. You'll also find links to products that not only don't work (such as homeopathy) but also can be actively dangerous (such as chelation therapy). Some of the instructions on the sites (dose your baby with vitamin C if he has whooping cough, for example) can directly endanger your baby's life if followed. If you choose to read the information on these websites, do so with extreme caution. Your child's life is too important to leave to ill-informed website creators and quacks with an agenda.

Those of us who understand the importance, safety, and efficacy of vaccines are often accused of using biased information and pushing medical science that does not work on an unsuspecting public. In truth, the information you'll find on pro-vaccine websites is often far more transparent and easy to trace. The same cannot be said about claims made on anti-vaccine websites. Many have links that do not work or argue the very opposite of what is claimed by the site. Many such sites also have funding sources that are not readily apparent.

Such sites often link to deeply flawed studies that have been debunked elsewhere. For example, most anti-vaccine websites continue to link to and use the now-discredited Wakefield study as their main source and justification. The sites that refer to this paper almost never mention the methodological flaws in the study, the discovered scientific fraud in the data, or the eventual retraction and repudiation of the study's results. If they mention the retraction at all, they claim it is the "medical establishment" persecuting Wakefield. Similarly, most anti-vaccine websites link to and use an article by Robert F. Kennedy Jr., originally published in the magazines *Rolling Stone* and *Salon*. That article, entitled "Deadly Immunity," was riddled with factual errors that required later correction. Eventually, the article was completely removed from both the *Rolling Stone* and *Salon* archives. The anti-vaccine websites that use this article rarely mention these corrections and retractions.

This list of anti-vaccine sites is not comprehensive, nor is it meant to be. These are merely some of the most visited anti-vaccine websites. Unfortunately, there are many others that have lots of bad information about vaccines. This list is our opinion and our opinion only. If you have any questions about any information you find on such sites, consult your pediatrician. *Never ever use the Internet as your sole source of medical information.*

Age of Autism Age of Autism is a website that calls itself "the nation's first daily Web newspaper for the environmental-biomedical community—those who believe autism is an environmentally-induced illness, that it is treatable, and that children can recover."[2] Unfortunately, only two of these claims are definitely true. Autism is treatable. A significant percentage of children initially diagnosed with autism can and do shake off the diagnosis eventually. A 2009 study by University of Connecticut professor Deborah Fein found that roughly 10 to 20 percent of all children diagnosed with autism were considered no longer autistic within several years after being diagnosed.[3] However, the claim that autism is environmentally induced is somewhat deceptive since the site focuses on only one possible environmental cause—vaccines.

Much of the site is devoted to making false allegations about vaccines. The discredited Dr. Andrew Wakefield is highly praised and fiercely defended. So is celebrity anti-vaccine activist Jenny McCarthy. The site also praises the retracted Robert F. Kennedy Jr. article. The authors mistakenly argue that vaccines cause everything from autism to arthritis to mercury poisoning to ADHD. The risks of vaccine-preventable diseases are largely ignored or vastly downplayed.

The site's authors also do a vast disservice to people with autism and their caregivers. They provide links to a long list of expensive products parents can buy to allegedly treat and even cure their children's illness. No scientific evidence exists to back up the claim that secretin or cod liver oil at over $12 a bottle will help them at all, let alone make their illness disappear. It is ironic that the authors of the site excoriate vaccine makers for making a small profit on an effective public health measure but unhesitatingly peddle much more profitable items that don't live up to their claims and may actually cause harm.

Mercola.com Dr. Joseph Mercola is an Illinois physician. Dr. Mercola claims to run "the world's #1 natural health website." This oft-quoted site contains a sad collection of quackery on many varied health topics, including cancer, allergies, and diabetes. His site contains a newsletter filled with all sorts of spurious allegations with no scientific support. His writings about vaccines are particularly inaccurate. According to Mercola, the hepatitis B vaccine can cause SIDS; Dr. Andrew Wakefield is right about measles and autism; and the flu vaccine can cause infertility. What should you do instead of using proven health measures that prevent infectious disease? Buy a home tanning bed! Take krill oil pills! Wash your hands with shea butter bar soap, and use moisturizing sweet orange bath and shower gel! All, of course, available for purchase on his website.

MotheringDotCommune MotheringDotCommune is the website of the now-defunct *Mothering* magazine, which ceased publication in 2011. The website is still, as of publication of this book, operating. The website does offer parents support for some excellent parenting practices such as nursing a baby for at least a year. However, this is drowned out by the pages and pages and pages of bad information presented by many posters as well as links to scientifically inaccurate articles from the *Mothering* archives. For example, site users are encouraged to give birth at home unattended even if they are at high risk of birthing complications. The section of the site devoted to vaccines is equally bad. Parents are urged to forgo nearly all vaccinations unless traveling overseas.

Users post unverified anecdotes of horrific vaccine reactions and deaths while downplaying the very real risk of vaccine-preventable diseases. Parents with babies who have whooping cough are told to stay away from medical professionals and simply "treat" the baby with massive doses of vitamins. Posters who attempt to provide scientifically valid information regarding vaccines are warned to cease and then banned if they persist. Their posts are censured and then erased. One of us was banned from the site for merely attempting to discuss the possibility that vaccinations are a valid parenting choice.

National Vaccine Information Center The National Vaccine Information Center (NVIC) is an organization founded by Barbara Loe Fisher, Jeff Schwartz, and Kathi Williams. NVIC calls itself "the oldest and largest consumer led organization advocating for the institution of vaccine safety and informed consent protections in the public health system."[4] The site entices parents with the assertion it is acting as a watch dog that will help them unearth the truth about vaccines.

Unfortunately NVIC is nothing of the sort. The site is filled with unverified and inaccurate information and links to highly misleading articles. For example, under the heading Diseases and Vaccines, you'll find a link labeled Diabetes. The implication is that vaccines cause diabetes, despite huge and well-documented studies indicating the contrary.[5] A similar link under the heading Polio/SV40 brings you to a link falsely indicating a possible connection between the polio vaccine and cancer. Both links lead to information that cites outdated or disproven studies, and neither provide the latest scientific research.

NVIC's authors repeatedly downplay the very real risk of vaccine-preventable diseases. Worse, the site's owners constantly imply there is a huge epidemic of vaccine injury and deaths of vaccine recipients that is deliberately being ignored by health officials who have been paid off by the pharmaceutical companies. Parents are urged to avoid vaccines and turn to ineffective alternatives such as homeopathy (which by definition is scientifically invalid) and chiropractic (which they claim can cure disease) instead. From a scientific standpoint, homeopathy involves reducing substances to make them stronger, often to dilutions that ensure that there is absolutely no active ingredient left. There is no current evidence for its effectiveness in preventing or curing disease beyond that of placebo. Chiropractic can be helpful for physical pain, but it cannot prevent disease the way vaccines do; there is no scientific evidence that chiropractic or homeopathy can substitute for vaccinating a child. Parents are also urged to explore Dr. Mercola's website; Mercola has supported the NVIC with donations, including a $1 million donation that the group indicates helped fund an anti-vaccine ad they posted on the Times Square Jumbotron that ran for weeks.[6]

A parent who reads the NVIC site can easily come away with the impression that she should skip certain vaccines or avoid vaccines altogether. In spite of the website's claims, that's not advocacy. That's disinformation.

ThinkTwice ThinkTwice is the online website of the New Atlantean Press. The site bills itself as a global vaccine institute. ThinkTwice has many sections including links to articles, books for sale by the publisher, an online support group, and a list of studies by supposedly reputable medical authorities.

The site is filled with allegations about government cover-ups and suggestions that vaccines aren't safe. Readers will find "evidence" of conspiracy theories such as the existence of a "Secret Government Database of Vaccine Damaged Children." The allegedly secret database? The VAERS (Vaccine Adverse Event Reporting System) database. As we point out in previous chapters, VAERS is not a secret. In fact, anyone can search it online at any time.

ThinkTwice leads readers to a list of scientific studies that are said to back up their anti-vaccine claims. The list is simply a recitation of studies without any way of allowing the reader to verify their contents. No links are provided to allow readers to check out the data independently. In some cases the authors of the site simply make an assertion and then provide no evidence at all to back up their claim. For example, the site claims a link between vaccines and SIDS (sudden infant death syndrome). The only evidence provided? A list of anecdotal e-mails and a link to an anti-vaccine book.

Whale.to Perhaps the Web's most notorious headquarters for every lunatic theory ever proposed, Whale is run by John Scudamore, an English pig farmer. If you've always wanted to read the anti-Semitic Czarist forgery *The Protocols of the Elders of Zion*, learn how CPR is a plot to control your children, or explore how the world is controlled by lizards, then this is the site for you.

Not surprisingly, Whale delves deeply into anti-vaccine propaganda. Dr. "Andy" Wakefield is quoted lovingly while parents are told to treat dangerous and infectious vaccine-preventable diseases with large doses of vitamin C.

The site is good for a laugh but not much else.

YOU'RE SMART—BE SMART
ABOUT YOUR INFORMATION SOURCES

Most parents are reasonably smart. Most of us can tell who is giving us information, for what purpose, and why. The motivations for a specific stance on this subject are fairly apparent. Yes, the online world can be enormous and quite confusing initially. But the obviously bad information is usually very obvious. All websites, indeed all writers, always have a bias. Most of us, including the writers of this book, come to the table with preconceived notions about ideas and people. The same is true of anyone who writes about anything, especially the subject of manufactured controversy such as vaccines.

But there's a huge difference between a group of scientists putting out accurate information backed by centuries of research and proven results and a few people getting together to put up a website. Always try to pull back the curtain to see what's really there. If you can't find that information, go elsewhere. If you find material that does not make sense or is proven wrong fairly easily, go elsewhere. A site put up by someone advocating homeopathy or selling products you know don't work as claimed should not have the same value to you as the website of the CDC. Most important of all, if you have a question about a vaccine, contact your doctor. The Internet should only serve as a secondary source of information. The CDC will help you find ways to comfort your child if she has a vaccine reaction. The NNii can help you decide if the latest vaccine makes sense for you and your children at the current time.

What the Web cannot do is be a substitute for your own good judgment. That is up to you. A 3:00 a.m. Web search is far less daunting for most people than a late-evening frantic call to a pediatrician. As long as you know where to look, the Internet can be a useful resource for information on this topic.

· *12* ·

Other Vaccine Myths and Facts

*N*o one source can answer every single question or concern you might have about vaccination. On any given day, hundreds of new Web pages are created. Some will inevitably contain confusing or misleading information about many topics including vaccination.

But certain myths about vaccines and vaccinations have cropped up over and over again on the Web. Some are merely silly or obviously hysterical. Others, however, may appear at first glance to contain a kernel of truth. Many anti-vaccine myths are propagated by very sincere people who, alas, are just plain wrong.

Here are some of those myths and the reality behind them.

THE AMISH DON'T VACCINATE AND DON'T GET AUTISM

Yes, they do, and yes, they do.

The Amish religion is a branch of Christianity that began in Switzerland in the seventeenth century. Since then, colonies of Amish have been established in many areas of the United States and Canada. Today most Amish shun many modern technologies including electricity and cars. The Amish work primarily as farmers and small businessmen in rural areas.

The origin of the myth regarding the Amish, vaccination, and autism probably stems from a single widely published article. In 2005, Dan Olmsted, a reporter for UPI and a regular contributor to the website Age of Autism, wrote a series of articles about his trips to Lancaster County, Pennsylvania. Lancaster is home to a large Amish community. Olmsted alleged that he'd gone looking for Amish people with autism and come up almost completely empty-handed. Why? Because, he implied, they vaccinated sparingly or refused vaccination altogether.

He was wrong on both counts.

Many Amish vaccinate, and many of them get autism. According to a report by the online magazine *Autism News Beat*, the Lancaster Amish community is home to the Clinic for Special Children (CSC). A reporter from the magazine made a call to the clinic and learned the following: "The idea that the Amish do not vaccinate their children is untrue," says Dr. Kevin Strauss, MD, a pediatrician at the CSC.[1] "We run a weekly vaccination clinic and it's very busy."[2] He says Amish vaccination rates are lower than the general population's, but younger Amish are more likely to be vaccinated than older generations.

Strauss also sees plenty of Amish children showing symptoms of autism.[3]

On several levels, none of this matters. The number of cases of autism in the Amish community ultimately tells us very little about the cause of autism or any potential links between vaccination and autism. The Amish are a largely genetically isolated community that can trace their roots back to a few hundred individuals. Even today most Amish people in the United States are descended from a small group of initial founders. As a result, their gene pool is different from the population as a whole. Certain rare diseases such as glutaric aciduria and maple syrup urine disease are far more common in the Amish community than the public at large.

Some Amish people have indeed chosen not to vaccinate their children. Unfortunately, their babies and children have repeatedly suffered as a result. In 2000, six unvaccinated Amish children died of Hib infection or meningitis in a single community.[4] Amish communities nationwide have coped with multiple outbreaks of vaccine-preventable diseases such as whooping cough, rubella, and chicken pox. In 2005, an Amish community was home to the first American cases of polio in twenty-six years.[5]

VACCINES ARE HUGELY PROFITABLE FOR THE PHARMACEUTICAL COMPANIES AND FOR DOCTORS

One of the most common assertions found on anti-vaccine websites is that vaccines are enormous moneymakers. A quick perusal of such websites yields headlines arguing that "profits, not science, motivate vaccine mandates!" Vaccines are said to be a multibillion-dollar business. Doctors, we are told, are in hock with pharmaceutical companies to foist vaccines on an unsuspecting public so both they and the companies can make money.

Let's take a closer look at this claim.

Most American vaccines are made by three companies today: Glaxo-SmithKline, Merck, and Sanofi Pasteur. In 1967, there were twenty-six companies manufacturing vaccines.[6] Why the decline? Because most vaccines really aren't that profitable. Certainly not when compared to other products, especially other pharmaceuticals.

Prevnar is the most profitable of all vaccines, with earnings of roughly a billion dollars each year.[7] Most vaccines aren't even close to making a tenth of that for manufacturers. Vaccines constitute only a very small part of an industry that sees nearly a trillion dollars in annual earnings.

Companies left the vaccine manufacturing business for a variety of reasons. These reasons include high liability potential, industry mergers, and greater research and development costs. Mostly they left because making vaccines was too costly and the potential for profit too low. Vaccines can be difficult to make. For example, each year vaccine makers prepare a new flu vaccine. They spend months trying to figure out exactly what particular strains are likely to be most dangerous that season. Then they spend money cultivating the material involved. Once the vaccine is on the market, the maker faces several risks including low demand and the fact that the vaccine expires. In 2010, a quarter of all flu vaccines were discarded because too much was produced in anticipation of an epidemic that never happened.[8]

Vaccines also have a smaller market than many other products. Some pharmaceuticals may be used for years or even a person's entire life. A single pill of Lipitor costs about $2 and must be taken every single day for maximum effect.[9] The measles, mumps, and rubella (MMR) shot costs less than $20 and is given only three times.[10] Not exactly big money by most standards.

Most vaccines are simply not huge moneymakers for the pharmaceutical companies. The companies would profit far more if people caught vaccine-preventable diseases instead. Before the MMR vaccine, just about all people caught measles. A significant percentage of them got sick enough to be hospitalized. The same would be true today if the MMR vaccine did not exist. Treating measles offers far more opportunities for profit than preventing it does.

Do you know what's really and truly expensive? Many alternative remedies. You can buy a "homeopathic accident and emergency kit" (basically distilled water) on Amazon for around $50. You could spend $75 and up for a single session of chelation therapy. This is the logic of the anti-vaccine movement. A small profit earned by vaccine makers for a product that works well is a sign of deep corruption in the vaccine industry. Much larger profits earned by products that don't work at all are not only not worthy of condemnation but actually deserve high praise.

You know what else is expensive? Outbreaks of vaccine-preventable diseases. A single person infected with measles in San Diego in 2008 led to twelve more cases. Health officials spent over $175,000 just to stop the spread of the disease.[11]

Overall, vaccines provide enormous benefits at very low cost. In the July 6, 2011, issue of the *Journal of the American Medical Association*, health officials estimated that vaccinations given from 2001 to 2010 saved over $83 billion in treatment and other related costs.[12] These vaccines saved roughly forty-two thousand lives, and twenty million fewer people were hospitalized.[13]

Any profit that vaccine makers make on vaccines is both well earned and well deserved. Vaccines are essential public health measures that work quite well. Some vaccines, such as the hepatitis B vaccine and the Gardasil vaccine, are known to prevent certain types of cancer. One in three of us will get cancer at some point in time.[14] A vaccine is one important action you can take to reduce your risk of certain types of cancers.

Even if pharmaceutical companies got out of the business of making vaccines, one fact would remain: vaccines are an essential cornerstone of public health. Someone has to make them. In the United States, they are manufactured largely by private industry, with some partnership with government agencies. In some countries, such as Denmark, vaccines are considered too important to be left to the whims of the free market. The government funds and controls the manufacturing process. However vaccine production is accomplished in a given country, the lack of such production would result in one thing—outbreaks of dangerous vaccine-preventable diseases.

After the breakup of the Soviet Union in the early 1990s, many Russian governmental departments failed to function effectively. As a result of this failure, many Russian children did not receive enough doses of the DTaP vaccine. Sadly, a diphtheria epidemic followed. The number of diphtheria cases in Russia jumped from 603 in 1989 to over 39,000 in 1994.[15] It took the combined efforts of several international health organizations including the Centers for Disease Control and Prevention (CDC) to finally get the epidemic under control.

Vaccination is one health measure that's both incredibly cheap and incredibly effective. We all save money when pharmaceutical companies make them.

GETTING THE DISEASE IS
BETTER THAN GETTING THE SHOT

Anti-vaccine groups often claim that getting an actual disease is far preferable to getting a vaccine. They assert that diseases such as measles, mumps, and even whooping cough may be unpleasant for a little while. But ultimately people will be healthier and stronger for having suffered through them. They argue that a bout of measles strengthens the immune system and provides immunity superior to the kind found in a shot.

None of these claims are true.

For one thing, getting a vaccine-preventable disease does not necessarily confer immunity. It may or it may not depending on the disease. For another, the cost of getting the disease is often very high. As documented in prior chapters, vaccine-preventable diseases often come with many potential side effects. A bout of mumps might leave a man sterile. A case of measles can lead to long-term hearing damage and even encephalitis. Measles is not exactly a fun experience for most people. Spending weeks in bed fighting off a serious illness does not make sufferers stronger in the short term or for the rest of their lives. Your immune system does not need such a vigorous workout to function properly.

In most cases, a shot is just as effective at providing immunity as getting the actual illness and certainly is far less painful. It is true that immunity against specific diseases may wear off over time if you get a shot. In that case, doctors recommend a booster shot. On the other hand, many vaccines, such as the MMR, confer lifelong immunity to most people. Both the pertussis disease and the pertussis vaccine provide protection for roughly ten years.[16] So even if you get pertussis itself and spend hours coughing so hard you gasp for air, you still face the possibility of getting the disease again, and your suffering was all for nothing. Certain diseases, such as tetanus, do not give you immunity once you've had them.[17] You could theoretically get tetanus several times. Some vaccine-preventable illnesses such as polio have multiple strains. In order to acquire natural immunity from polio you would need to come down with the disease more than once.

Without vaccines, most people, instead of getting a few shots, would come down with at least several vaccine-preventable diseases. Every single time you would get a disease, you'd face huge risks and a long recovery period. Worse, most people would get such illnesses as young babies or children when they are most vulnerable to disease complications.

THE HEPATITIS B VACCINE CAUSES SIDS

The hepatitis B vaccine is given shortly after birth to help prevent babies from getting this form of hepatitis. Hepatitis in young children does all sorts of nasty things. Many cases will lead to liver failure because little kids are unable to clear the infection as effectively as their adult counterparts.

Critics allege the vaccine is unnecessary. Sometimes, they go further and argue it can actually cause children to die from sudden infant death syndrome (SIDS). SIDS is an ancient baby killer. A small infant will suddenly die during the night without any apparent cause. Theories abound as to what can trigger SIDS. Scientists are still not quite sure. The leading proven method of prevention is to lay a baby on her back when she's sleeping. Increased use of this technique has led to a huge reduction in the number of deaths from SIDS in the last several decades.

The use of the hepatitis B vaccine has not been correlated with an increase in the number of SIDS cases. For example, in 1992 only 8 percent of all infants were given the hepatitis B vaccine.[18] This was the first year the vaccine was recommended to all parents. During that year, the U.S. Department of Health and Human Services reported 4,800 SIDS deaths.[19] By 1996, vaccine usage had increased to 82 percent of all babies.[20] If the hepatitis B vaccine really were a risk factor for SIDS, one would expect to see a corresponding increase in the number of SIDS deaths. Yet the number of SIDS cases actually fell to 3,000 during that year.[21]

Similar numbers have been reported since the vaccine has been in use. The number of SIDS cases fluctuates from year to year without any correlation to the number of hepatitis B vaccines used.

There's no evidence whatsoever to back up this false assertion.

DISEASES DISAPPEARED BECAUSE OF BETTER HYGIENE, NOT VACCINES

Most Americans no longer think about a lot of diseases you can still find in much of the developing world. Very few Americans have even heard of cholera, let alone ever seen a case of it. The same is true of many diseases you'll find in the history books, such as scarlet fever and dysentery. Tuberculosis, once the scourge of Europe, has largely been eliminated in many European countries even as it remains a serious problem in much of Asia.

Why?

Better sanitation. It is true that clean water and access to effective sanitation can reduce the instances of many diseases. Without it such diseases can easily come back. In 2010, a devastating earthquake struck Haiti. One of the troubling aftermaths of this natural disaster has been outbreaks of cholera. We don't get cholera in the United States or other developed nations, basically because we don't have poop in our drinking water.

The discovery of antibiotics has also saved countless lives. For example, scarlet fever is a very bad form of strep throat. Today patients are treated with antibiotics before it gets that far. The disease still appears in some places occasionally. In 2011, nearly a thousand Chinese people came down with it.[22]

Clean water, effective sanitation, and antibiotics are truly modern inventions too often taken for granted unless you've spent lots of time in a developing country. But they are only half the story.

Vaccines are the other half.

Take a look at some of the most recent vaccines. The Hib vaccine protects against a virulent form of meningitis. The vaccine to prevent Hib was not introduced until the late 1980s. Since that time, the number of deaths and infections from Hib has fallen drastically. Have we magically gotten cleaner since that time? Are we washing our hands more? Has American sanitation improved in the last twenty years? Of course not.

The only thing that reduced the number of Hib cases has been the vaccine. Before the Hib vaccine more than twenty thousand babies got Hib each year.[23] By 2002 that number had fallen to thirty-four cases.[24] The same is true of many other vaccines. The MMR vaccine was not developed until the early 1970s. Indoor plumbing was a standard part of nearly all American housing by the 1920s. That did not stop mortality rates from measles. The vaccine did. Vincent Astor was one of the richest men of his day. In 1914, shortly after he married, he came down with mumps. As a result, Astor became sterile. Astor was not a victim of bad plumbing or poor hygiene. His misfortune was just another result of the era before vaccines.

You can clean your house six times a day. You can breastfeed your children until they're trying out for the football team. You can eat only organic, use cloth diapers, and practice attachment parenting until your baby wears out a dozen Snuglis. None of this will protect your baby, toddler, or child the same way his series of shots will.

YOU SHOULD SPREAD VACCINES OUT OR DELAY THEM

Some anti-vaccine websites claim that vaccines should be more widely spaced out than the current schedule. They tell parents to defer vaccines until the child's immune system is better developed. They also advocate that parents break up shots and give fewer on each pediatric visit. So instead of giving an MMR shot, the anti-vaccine movement urges parents to give a separate measles, mumps, and rubella vaccines at different pediatric visits.

The anti-vaccine movement claims that spreading out vaccines and delaying them offers several advantages. They argue that spreading out vaccines allows parents to better monitor any potential vaccine reactions and find out which particular vaccine is causing a reaction. They also suggest that doing so means less stress on an infant's body.

This is faulty reasoning on multiple fronts. The American vaccine schedule, like those found in other countries, isn't picked out of a hat. Many health authorities contribute to development of the recommended schedule. The timing of any new vaccine is carefully considered by the American Academy of Pediatrics, the Centers for Disease Control and Prevention, and the American Academy of Family Physicians. Some vaccines are given earlier or later depending on the ability of the baby's immune system to fully absorb the vaccine's intended effects. The medical experts don't sit around and decide the details of the schedule by throwing darts at it.

For instance, the first dose of the hepatitis B vaccine is given within a few hours of birth. The vaccine is given at this time because studies show that babies are able to gain protection from the disease even at this young age. Other vaccines, such as the MMR, are given later as the baby grows because immunity may not take if given any earlier. Randomly deciding when to give a specific vaccine ignores the scientific reasons vaccines are given at a certain age.

Delaying vaccines does not reduce the possibility of a vaccine reaction. A baby is just as likely to react to a vaccine if you give that vaccine at six months or when the child is two. Delaying vaccines also does not decrease the possibility that the child will have a serious problem from the vaccine. Health investigators have examined this issue very closely. A study published in the June 1, 2010, issue of *Pediatrics* looked at the vaccination records of more than a thousand kids. Researchers at the University of Louisville found no evidence that delaying vaccines improved neurophysical development.[25]

The only thing delaying vaccines accomplishes is to increase the risk your baby or child may get a vaccine-preventable disease. Many vaccine-preventable diseases are more dangerous for younger children. An adult may find a bout of whooping cough irritating. A young baby faces all kinds of serious risks from the same disease, including brain damage and death.

Even if you decide to vaccinate later or wait until after you hear about an outbreak, it can take up to two weeks for certain vaccines to work. In the meantime, your child remains at risk. A delayed schedule also means more shots later on when a child is older and her fears are less easily soothed. A young baby, unlike older children, can be nursed as she is given her shots and thus provided with a form of comfort to help immediately alleviate any pain. This is more difficult to accomplish with an older child.

Breaking up vaccines into individual components is also not a good idea. Breaking up the MMR vaccine actually means two more shots than necessary, thus two more pediatrician visits and two more chances to upset your child. In addition, if the anti-vaccine movement is concerned about exposing children to the ingredients in vaccines, more shots means more exposure. Why would they advocate for that? Finally, although serious vaccine reactions are highly unlikely in the first place, more shots means more chances for this unlikely event to occur.

There are legitimate reasons to delay or skip vaccinations. A premature baby may not be ready for certain vaccines. A toddler might have a bad reaction to a specific vaccine, so his doctor may recommend against further dosages. But parents should not skip or delay vaccinations unless specifically told to do so by their child's pediatrician. The risks of doing so outweigh any alleged benefits.

CERTAIN COUNTRIES DO NOT USE VACCINES

Or they use alternative schedules or don't use certain vaccines. This myth contains a tiny bit of truth. Nearly all countries use vaccines. Those that skip many vaccines do so because the countries in question often have health budgets so small they cannot afford even the nominal cost of most vaccines. Vaccine usage is coordinated and supervised by the governing health body of each individual nation. Thus, the American vaccination schedule can differ quite a bit from that of other countries. In many developing nations, access to vaccines is very limited. Even in more developed nations, the kind of vaccines used can differ vastly from nation to nation.

Health officials may also decide against specific vaccines for a period of time and then go back to using them. These decisions can have awful consequences. From 2003 to 2009, Nigerian government officials essentially stopped using the polio vaccine. Why? Because religious extremists preached that the vaccine was a plot designed by Westerners to harm Nigerian girls. The result sparked a worldwide resurgence of polio. The disease quickly spread to other nearby nations and then to countries outside of Africa. Polio was once nearly the second disease to be completely eradicated by vaccination. Unfortunately, as of this writing and solely because of the scaremongering tactics used in Nigeria, the disease remains a public health problem in several countries.

Similar problems arose in Sweden with the pertussis vaccine. A vaccine for whooping cough was introduced in the 1950s. The vaccine worked.

Whooping cough cases fell by two-thirds.[26] Unfortunately, an influential Swedish medical leader presented a paper arguing that the vaccine was not necessary and was not responsible for this decline. After media attention to his false claims, the pertussis vaccination rate in Sweden fell drastically.

The result was quite predictable. Widespread use of the vaccine had pushed Swedish pertussis rates down from three hundred out of a hundred thousand to fifty out of a hundred thousand.[26] When vaccination rates dropped, whooping cough rates began to climb again. Within the next ten years, six out of every ten Swedish children got sick with whooping cough.[27] More than two thousand children were hospitalized, and more than fifty were permanently disabled.[28] In 1996, the Swedes started to use the whooping cough vaccine again.[29] The rates of pertussis have declined dramatically as a result.

The Japanese also got caught up in the anti–whooping cough vaccine fallacy. Their children suffered greatly because of it. Pertussis vaccination rates declined from 80 percent to 10 percent in the space of two years.[30] Forty-one children died needlessly because they were not vaccinated against whooping cough until officials decided to return to the vaccine in 1981.[31] Since that time, the vaccine has gained acceptance in Japan. As a result the number of cases of whooping cough has fallen enormously.

VACCINES ARE CONTROVERSIAL

Opposition to vaccination is nothing new. Anti-vaccine protests have been around since the introduction of smallpox variolation. As each new development in vaccination technology has appeared, people have continued to argue against vaccination and the principles behind it. This historical trend continues to haunt us today.

It is easy to fear vaccination. The very idea that an injection of a killed virus can protect you against an actual disease does not seem to make sense initially. Needles are very scary things. Yet when looked at carefully and logically, the principles behind the science of vaccines are not that difficult to grasp.

The anti-vaccine movement has made several arguments against vaccination. Their primary assertions are that the safety and efficacy of inoculations are in dispute; the science of vaccines isn't clear; and even at present, health officials regard vaccination as a controversial procedure fraught with risk.

These arguments are completely and utterly untrue.

The science behind vaccination is not under dispute. The mechanisms by which vaccines work will not be a source of contention in college classes in chemistry or biology. It is true some of the more esoteric mechanisms of vaccine-induced immunity are the subject of ongoing research by scientists and discussion by interested observers. But essential and basic vaccination principles such as herd immunity, antigens, booster shots, and the ability of the body to manufacture antibodies are not in doubt and never have been.

There's so much we don't know about the human body. Scientists still aren't sure how to cure the common cold. Researchers don't know how to make us all live to be 110. They're not even sure why some people live to be 110. The fundamental principles of the universe elude us. We have yet to travel to the nearest star or even the nearest planet. The bottom of the sea remains as uncharted as the planets circling distant stars.

The same cannot be said of vaccines. Vaccination is an established technology dating back hundreds of years. Very few medical procedures have the same documented history as inoculation does. We know vaccines work. We mostly know how they work. We know how to make vaccines that prevent many diseases, lower infant mortality rates, and reduce the effects even if you get sick. We know how to give you a single shot or a series of shots that would allow nearly all people to walk into a room full of measles germs and leave without getting infected.

We know that if you don't give babies vaccines, they'll be at serious risk of all kinds of diseases that can ruin their hearing, eyesight, and brains. We know that children who cannot be vaccinated because of an underlying medical condition benefit when others are vaccinated. No reputable pediatrician will tell a parent anything else.

Anti-vaccine activists can try to imply otherwise, but they still can't change the fundamental facts about this issue.

Vaccines work. Pointing that out—and demanding that we continue to vaccinate—is the best way to honor the work done by those engaged in the difficult field of medical research.

· *13* ·

Modern Developments in Vaccine Technology: The Story of the HPV Vaccine

$\mathcal{V}$accine development is an ever-changing field. The science of vaccines is built on fundamental known principles. Vaccines are constantly being monitored for efficacy and modified as needed. Unlike anti-vaccine activists who cling to discredited theories even when massive evidence indicates such theories are wrong, scientists routinely discard ideas that don't work. New research results allow scientists to understand how to make old vaccines better. This new information also allows for the development of new vaccines for diseases that always haunted humanity.

Two of the most recently developed vaccines protect against the human papillomavirus (HPV). These vaccines draw on both old and new ideas. HPV contributes to the development of certain cancers.[1,2,3] Both vaccines are the latest target of the anti-vaccine propaganda. They are also controversial because HPV is a sexually transmitted disease.[4] Many parents are reluctant to think about their children's future sexual behavior. This reluctance can lead them to delay or avoid giving their children the HPV vaccine.

HPV—SILENT, SOMETIMES DEADLY

Scientists have identified between one hundred and two hundred strains of HPV. About forty of them are sexually transmitted.[5] The majority of these infections do not cause any obvious symptoms. Therefore, most people who have the virus are unaware they are infected. Most of the sexually transmitted HPV strains are benign, and the infections resolve naturally with no long-term damage.[6] However, a small percentage of the strains is associated with

147

genital warts in both men and women.[7,8] Some of the strains of HPV are also associated with various types of precancerous and cancerous conditions. HPV has been implicated in the vast majority of cervical cancers[9] as well as penile cancers, anal cancers, and cancers of the throat and tonsils.[10,11]

Cervical cancer in women starts out with a condition known as dysplasia, in which abnormal cells grow on the surface of the cervix. Most dysplasias are detected through routine Pap smears and treated early enough to prevent the condition from advancing. Treatment for cervical dysplasia involves removing the abnormal cell growths through a variety of methods. This treatment may interfere with pregnancy later in the woman's life, including possibly leaving women unable to successfully bear children.[12]

Undetected or unmonitored dysplasia can advance to cervical cancer. This type of cancer has few symptoms. Most of those symptoms occur after the cancer has spread to other organ systems, making successful treatment difficult. Treatment for cervical cancer includes surgical removal of the cervix, uterus, and possibly the ovaries. All of this means the woman will not be able to have children. If cancer cells have spread from the cervix to other parts of the body, treatment may also include radiation or chemotherapy. Cervical cancer kills about four thousand women in the United States[13] and about two hundred thousand women worldwide every year.[14]

In the United States, penile cancer is diagnosed in approximately thirteen hundred men each year, and approximately three hundred men die each year.[15] As with cervical cancer, penile cancer also has few symptoms. Treatment involves removal of the abnormal cells,[16,17] sometimes requiring removal of the entire penis.[17] If the cancer has spread to other parts of the body, other treatments such as chemotherapy may be required.

The CDC estimates that twenty million Americans carry HPV infection.[18] Many of those Americans are unaware they are infected. Infection by the HPV strains associated most with cervical cancer in women and penile cancer in men can be prevented by vaccination.

GARDASIL AND CERVARIX

Two vaccines are currently available to help HPV infection: Gardsasil, marketed by Merck, and Cervarix, marketed by GlaxoSmithKline. The work on Gardasil began in the 1980s. The first phase of development involved research that utilized the gold standard of experimental methodology—the double-blind design. A double-blind design is the most controlled, most valid form of experiment available. Whenever possible, scientists attempt to use that design to test hypotheses.

When testing a new drug, researchers randomly sample the population they are studying. They then randomly assign that sample to at least two different groups. One group will receive the actual drug being tested (the experimental group), and the other group (the control group) will receive an inactive substance (a placebo). In a double-blind design, neither the people administrating the dose nor the people receiving the dose know whether they are receiving the actual drug. This allows researchers to control for the placebo effect. This effect occurs when people get better or don't get sick because they believe they won't get sick, not because of an actual drug. A double-blind design also prevents the researchers from unconsciously or consciously biasing their data in support of their drug. This ensures that any differences in the results between the two groups are actually because of the drug.

This experimental method was used in the original development phase of both Gardasil and Cervarix. In the initial development phase for Gardasil, more than twelve thousand young women ages sixteen to twenty-six from thirteen countries were randomly chosen to participate. After those women gave their consent, they were randomly assigned to receive either the experimental vaccine or a placebo vaccine.[19] The rates of HPV infection in the experimental group were so significantly decreased that the research was ended early so all the young women could receive the vaccine.[20] Ending an experiment of this type early is a rare occurrence in research. However, scientists felt it was unethical to keep it from the placebo group since the results indicated it worked so well.

Gardasil is not effective against an existing HPV infection. It is not as effective in women older than twenty-six.[21] It is most effective, therefore, when given to women prior to their becoming sexually active and thus running the risk of being infected without their knowledge. It protects against four strains of HPV known to be associated with cervical dysplasia and cancer. The vaccine uses virus-like particles made up of proteins from those virus strains, not whole viruses. It is administered in three doses over a six-month period.[22]

Cervarix's development process was similar. It was tested in two phases. The first phase involved more than a thousand American women. The second phase involved over eighteen thousand women from fourteen countries. The design of both these phases was also double blind and randomized. Cervarix protects against two strains of HPV and uses virus-like particles of those strains.[23] Neither Cervarix nor Gardasil contain thimerosal.

Gardasil is often preferred by medical authorities and public health officials since it protects against four strains of HPV. Both vaccines are recommended for both men and women, as they protect against reproductive cancers for both sexes. Vaccinating men and women also increases herd immunity against HPV. Because the research regarding the use of Gardasil for men is relatively new, however, the focus of public policy is the vaccination of girls.

Almost immediately, these vaccines became the focus of political and medical controversy. The first criticism of the vaccine came from conservative religious sources. Both the Family Research Council[24] and Focus on the Family made public statements that allowing young women to receive the vaccine would increase sexual promiscuity. The fear of a sexually transmitted disease was considered by these groups to be an important deterrent to adolescent and premarital sexual intercourse. Of course, these statements ignore the fact it is possible even for married people to pass an HPV infection to their partners. Most HPV infections are asymptomatic. Even when the infections are symptomatic, those symptoms can show up years after the initial infection. Later, reports from these organizations stated they were not against the vaccine but against making it mandatory.

After the introduction of Gardasil, Merck began to lobby members of Congress to require the vaccination for eleven- and twelve-year-old girls before they would be allowed to attend school. Medical doctors pointed out that mandatory vaccination was more appropriate for diseases spread through casual contact. The HPV strains that Gardasil protects against are passed only through sexual contact. Merck dropped their campaign soon afterward.[25] Unfortunately this campaign helped fuel anti-vaccine conspiracy theories about vaccine manufacturers' intentions.

Proposals in most states to make the vaccine mandatory were not successful. In 2007, Texas governor and eventual 2012 Republican presidential candidate Rick Perry did issue an executive order mandating that girls be vaccinated.[26] The Texas legislature later overturned this order.[27] As of the writing of this book, the vaccine is mandatory only in Virginia and the District of Columbia. However both of these have opt-out programs.

The most pervasive controversy regarding Gardasil involves familiar accusations of dangerous reactions to the vaccine. The anti-vaccine movement reports that many thousands of young women are experiencing adverse reactions, and those reactions are going unreported or being underreported by medical authorities. The reported reactions range from fainting or dizziness all the way through death. Another 2012 Republican presidential candidate Michele Bachmann stated after her debate appearances that she'd received reports the shot caused mental retardation in one recipient.[28] She did not provide identifying information of this supposed victim. Bioethicist Art Caplan offered $10,000 for proof of this claim.[29] The money has never been claimed. Representative Bachmann stated in a subsequent campaign event that recipients of the vaccine were having to endure "the ravages" caused by it.[30] She offered no evidence for this statement.

Like many reports of adverse effects from other vaccines, these reports about the HPV vaccine are problematic for a couple of reasons. First, the administration of both the Gardasil and the Cervarix vaccine takes place in three shots over a six-month period. A great deal can happen during six months. If a young woman has a seizure during the period of time between the first and second or second and third dose, is that seizure due to the vaccine? According to the anti-vaccine movement, yes. The problem with assuming that every medical condition that occurs during a vaccination schedule is due to vaccines is again a problem of timing. How can such a determination be made? By the use of double-blind randomized experimental research. The development phases of both the Gardasil and Cervarix vaccines used such a model and found no statistically significant differences in adverse reactions between the groups of women receiving the vaccines and the groups of women receiving the placebo. They certainly did not find any instances of paralysis, mental retardation, or death, as is being reported by the anti-vaccine movement. In addition, a follow-up study of 380,000 shots found 35 severe reactions in that sample, a reaction rate of 0.009 percent.[31] A second follow-up study found a rate of severe allergic reaction of 2.6 out of 100,000 doses.[32]

A second issue with such reports of adverse effects is that many of the people and anti-vaccine groups making those statements, such as Barbara Loe Fisher of the National Vaccine Information Center,[33] are relying on the VAERS database for their "proof." As we've discussed already, using the VAERS in this way is inappropriate. The data in question is unverified until investigated further. Statements of causality—that one thing causes another—cannot be made when referring to reports in the VAERS.

On the surface, some of the reports floating around about the Gardasil vaccine may appear to be quite startling. In the last few years, dozens of reports of deaths related to the Gardasil vaccine have been entered into the VAERS. Anti-vaccine activists have seized on these reports as evidence that Gardasil not only does not work as advertised but is actually killing off young women.

The real data, when examined more closely, very clearly points to the contrary. According to Merck's own statement during the Gardasil trials "across the clinical studies, 17 deaths were reported in 21,464 male and female subjects."[34] Seventeen deaths sounds like a lot when you first hear it. Yet of those seventeen, four were from automobile accidents. Vaccines obviously do not cause car accidents. In fact, as we pointed out previously, children are more in danger from a car accident on the way to the pediatrician's office than they are from any shot. Additional causes of death listed are from suicide/overdose, sepsis, and asphyxia. Again this is consistent with what we can expect to find in normal patterns at this age. Adolescent girls use drugs. They suffer from mental illnesses that lead to successful suicide attempts. This will happen with or without the vaccine.[35]

Additional reports of death can be found in the VAERS database after the vaccine was released and used in the general population. They can also be dated to a certain time frame. If you look at the listings up to August 2009, you will find thirty-two additional reports of deaths there. Again a close look at the causes of death is fully consistent with what we would expect to find in this population had the vaccine not been administered. Listed causes of death include blood clots, diabetes, and seizure disorders.[36] The girls in question had other risk factors such as smoking and use of oral contraceptives that can be ruled in as probable cause of the deaths. In any given year we can unfortunately expect to see young women dying from a variety of causes including smoking while using birth control pills and poorly controlled diabetes. A great deal of evidence indicates that use of the Gardasil vaccine is not one of those causes.

More than ten million people have received the vaccine since it became available. This is a huge number of people. It is certainly enough to confidently assert that any legitimate pattern of severe adverse reactions would have been identified and addressed by now. After all, the original rotavirus vaccine was pulled and revamped due to patterns of reactions identified from VAERS reports.

The fact that girls and boys should be vaccinated against HPV before they become sexually active means the best time for this vaccination is as early as possible, preferably prior to thirteen years of age. Many parents find the idea of vaccinating their young child against a potential future sexually transmitted disease to be distasteful. As a parent, it's normal to be uncomfortable when thinking about the future sexual behavior of your children. This discomfort should not prevent you from making the right decision for your children by making sure they receive the HPV vaccine as recommended, nor should it make you worry once your children have gotten the vaccine.

The vaccine for HPV is an example of how doctors are using old vaccine technology to combat new diseases. It is also an example of how anti-vaccine foes have continued to distort information, bombard parents with false data, and create controversy where there is none to be found. Health officials studied the issue for years, discovered a solution, and tested it thoroughly. The vaccine has been offered to the public. We have tremendous evidence that it works as promised. Evidence gathered in a short amount of time indicates the vaccine will help greatly lower the number of cases of cervical cancer and help women live longer and healthier lives. Australia was the very first nation to fund the vaccine in 2007.[37] Since then, researchers have already found evidence of a drop in the number of HPV infections and a corresponding reduction in high-grade cervical abnormalities in Australian women who have received the HPV vaccine.[38]

Better hygiene did not reduce the number of precancerous lesions in young Australian girls. Organic food is not the reason they will see fewer scary Pap smears or have a lower chance of dealing with genital warts. The vaccine did that in a few short years.

The HPV vaccine may be particularly important in the developing world. According to the National Cancer Coalition, 85 percent of all cervical cancer cases occur in less developed countries.[39] Many women in these countries do not have access to annual Pap smears. Use of the vaccine has the potential to drastically reduce the number of annual deaths even in the absence of access to basic medical care.

This is one of the ultimate legacies of a centuries-old technology. That we can take techniques known to us for hundreds of years, refine them, and use them to help us today is astonishing. We can still use old vaccines to prevent disease by refining them, improving them, and making them even better than ever. We can also create new vaccines. As of this writing, researchers are investigating vaccines against dozens of diseases including cancer, HIV, cholera, dengue fever, malaria, and Staph-resistant infections. The current vaccine schedule may be greatly expanded one day. Rather than enduring painful diseases, people may be able to simply line up periodically for a patch that rests against the skin or a thin stream of air that presses into your neck and provides lifelong protection against multiple illnesses.

The Easiest Parenting
Decision You'll Make

 $\mathcal{S}$ ince the days of Edward Jenner, every parent has been forced to grapple with the issue of vaccines in one way or another. Walk back in time a few centuries and you will hear the same questions about this issue as you would today. The alleged debate over vaccines is not new. In some ways it is the oldest of all debates: the issue of very minor individual risk versus wider public health considerations has been with us since people came together in groups larger than two. People have always sought to figure out what is best for all while minimizing risks to each person. From the days of the Roman Senate to parliamentary debates to the speaker on the corner soapbox to the local newspaper, public health has always been a subject of fierce and often hot and loud debate.

The very same websites that accuse pharmaceutical companies of being in league with the government to poison children are the direct offshoots of the same protestors who marched through the streets holding an effigy of Edward Jenner. Jenny McCarthy's assertions that vaccines caused her son's autism mirror the assertions of people in the 1800s who insisted that vaccination against smallpox would cause people to turn into pigs.

Fear of vaccination is one of our oldest fears.

Such fears are understandable. Vaccination has always seemed somewhat counterintuitive to most people. Why would you knowingly inject a baby with infectious material that has the potential to cause harm? Why would you not wait until your newborn is a bit older and less vulnerable?

At the same time a quick scan of most historic texts tells us the opposite story. Measles, smallpox, diphtheria, and half a dozen other illnesses stalk across the world stage and drag people off with them to an agonizing death. Many people today can recall hours spent itching from chicken pox or tales of relatives seriously affected by polio. A family tree project often leads into branches with relatives who died very young of diseases that are clearly preventable today.

So on the surface the issue initially appears quite complex for many people. Do your own research, believe in your own instincts, and remember you know what's best for your child, exhort the anti-vaccine activists. You have the freedom to decide. You should not be coerced into a decision with possibly life-threatening complications that could have serious and long-term side effects.

They are right.

You should research and believe in your own instincts. You should have the freedom to decide what to do and the understanding of what happens when you make a choice on this issue. All parents should have some understanding of each vaccine and the diseases they help prevent. All parents should understand basic terms used by medical professionals about this issue. That includes ideas such as herd immunity, antigens, and booster shots. You should know what each vaccine ingredient does as well as the risks of receiving shots instead of getting the diseases they help prevent. All parents should feel comfortable talking to their pediatricians and confident they can ask appropriate questions.

What parents shouldn't do is panic. They shouldn't fear or run away from vaccines. Vaccination is a fairly straightforward issue that has been understood for several hundred years. Vaccines use the body's own immune system to help it fight off potentially serious diseases. If everyone or nearly everyone vaccinates, vaccine-preventable diseases cannot take hold in any given population. Essentially we're using a weakened form of many bad diseases in order to stop them from infecting anyone.

The results of vaccination programs are very obviously and easily seen. No one in the entire world has died from smallpox in several decades. Our babies are not deaf from congenital rubella syndrome. They aren't paralyzed by polio or mentally impaired from Hib. American parents do not worry their children's throats will swell up from mumps or look carefully for the telltale Koplik's spots that bode an onset of measles.

In countries where people don't use vaccines, the results are equally obvious. As of this writing, hundreds of thousands of children in India die each year simply because they have not been vaccinated against measles. Hib and neonatal tetanus still steal the lives of thousands of children in Asia and Africa. In areas where people willfully refuse vaccination, the diseases don't just go away. In 2011, more than fifteen thousand people in France came down with measles. Six people died from a totally preventable disease.[1]

These facts are not under dispute. The availability of the vacuum cleaner and the use of the dishwasher did not stop polio or mumps. Martha Stewart herself cannot prevent tetanus, nor can organic foods reduce the contagiousness of the flu. The diseases in question are not under dispute either. Without vaccination efforts such diseases will be back. Mumps is not going to go away because you don't think it poses a problem. The whooping cough bacterium isn't any less dangerous because you've been using cloth instead of disposable diapers.

The anti-vaccine contingent tries to poke holes in these arguments at every turn. It's understandable that parents listen to them. A well-done website can look very convincing when Google leads you there at three in the morning after your baby daughter's measles, mumps, and rubella (MMR) shot. The links on your aunt's Facebook page sound fine when your cousins explain them to you over the phone.

What we hope this book does is give you the tools to understand what you need to know about this issue. As you have seen throughout this book, it's quite easy to become overwhelmed and confused by the amount of data out there. The process of deciding to vaccinate your child is made that much more difficult when the anti-vaccine movement is shouting (mostly) inaccurate information from the rooftops while scientists are quietly proving that vaccines are safe and effective.

We've aimed to give you a background in the basic medical facts about vaccines so you can understand why they work. We've also tried to explore the history of vaccination efforts and the risks surrounding both vaccination and vaccine-preventable diseases. We've shown that regardless of the time or vaccine, there have always been opponents to the technology, both reasonable and unreasonable.

We've given you statistics on the numbers of deaths caused by various vaccine-preventable diseases, both prior to vaccines and after vaccines. We've shown you a snapshot of what life was like for parents and children prior to the development of vaccines. That snapshot indicates just how important vaccines are to your child specifically and to public health in general.

We've explained what ingredients are in the most common vaccines, what they do, and why they're used. We've put those ingredients in perspective for you so you'll understand the amounts are minuscule and are used for scientific reasons. We've differentiated between real, established (and rare) vaccine reactions and unfounded accusations of reactions.

We've debunked the most widely misunderstood study linking vaccines with autism. We summarized why that study was misleading from the start and how the media perpetuated the hoax. This particular study is the main reason parents express doubts about vaccines, and now you know why the study was fraudulent and unreliable. We've also identified a few of the most vocal and well-known members of the anti-vaccine movement and explained why their information is invalid. We've given you tools to find information and separate out the good, the bad, and the horribly inaccurate.

In short, we hope we've given you much of what you need to know about this issue. We also hope we've shown you where to look for more information about this topic when the baby's crying at dawn and you don't want to wake up the nice pediatrician with yet more questions.

Ultimately, we feel this issue can be confusing, but it is not difficult to understand. Most babies and children should be vaccinated on time and according to the accepted pediatric schedule. Doing so offers both them and the rest of the population our best protection against many serious childhood diseases. Babies should forgo vaccinations only for medical reasons. Such reasons should be carefully explored with the help of your child's doctor. If such children can be safely given shots later in life, they should be vaccinated. Refusing vaccinations for a healthy child who can be vaccinated is not a good idea. Loudly proclaiming one's opposition to vaccination after refusing it is an even more rash and foolish course of action.

Let's face it.

Although being a parent is often a joyous and pleasant task, it is also one of life's hardest assignments. Parenting is a very hard job if done right. From nearly the very moment of conception, the worry clock begins ticking. Many an expectant mother frets over the many possible things that can go wrong with her baby. She worries she isn't eating right during her pregnancy and that she's gained too much or too little weight and this may influence her baby badly. Once labor begins, women confront the possibility that an epidural or C-section may cause difficulties for her infant. As her child grows, she may worry about using formula rather than breast milk, putting a baby in daycare, and choosing a good preschool. As her baby becomes a child, more worries pop up. Parenting means worrying about a child's grades. It means being scared your child is eating too much or too little. It means the nagging thought that your child isn't doing his homework properly, making enough friends, and doing enough to prepare himself for life after he leaves childhood behind.

Vaccinations are the one parenting decision that should not come with worry. Unlike teaching a child how to cope with a bully or pass algebra, the decision to vaccinate against pertussis, Hib, measles, and eleven other illnesses on the schedule is easy. No one—not Hollywood starlets, doctors, neighbors, relatives, politicians, or fellow parents—should ever make that decision harder. In addition, no one should put an entire community at risk of horrible diseases out of ignorance or fear.

Vaccines are, and always will be, the one decision just about every parent can understand fully. Much of the science is often unclear about many other major parenting decisions. Breastfeeding is probably better for a baby than formula. But most babies will survive and even thrive on formula. Some babies would die without access to formula as they are unable to digest breast milk. A few hours a day in daycare may or may not be better for your child than a bored mother and a family that lacks enough income to afford basic essential necessities. A good preschool is a useful foundation that can help prepare your child for life, but experts are not in agreement over what makes a good preschool or even a good elementary school effective.

Experts are sure of one single parenting decision. That decision is vaccination. Vaccines greatly increase the odds your baby will not get sick from more than a dozen pretty awful diseases. Anyone who implies the contrary does all parents a vast disservice.

In a world that often seems overloaded with difficult and contradictory information, we hope we've provided you with a lot of useful information on this subject. We hope you will walk away from this book not only knowing that vaccination is the right decision for just about all babies and children but also knowing why. We hope that by reading this book, you'll not only understand vaccination better but also discover where to find additional answers for any questions you may have.

Most of all we hope you will feel more confident about your decision to vaccinate. The lady with stage-four breast cancer down the block, the elderly woman who lives alone and takes five medications a day, the little girl who really did have a nasty reaction to her DTaP shot and cannot get any more vaccines—all of them depend on you and your choices.

Vaccinate your children. Do so knowing you are protecting them, their community, and even future generations who may one day add to the wondrous list of vaccine-vanquished diseases. Do so confidently, knowing you are making the best possible choice for your community and your children.

Notes

CHAPTER 2

1. T. C. Eickhorn. (2008). Penicillin: An accidental discovery changed the course of medicine. *Endocrine Today*. Retrieved from www.endocrinetoday.com/view.aspx ?rid=30176

2. World Health Organization. (2006, July 10). About WHO. Retrieved from https://apps.who.int/aboutwho/en/achievements.html

3. Ibid.

4. S. Downshen. (2009, November). Smallpox. Retrieved from http://kidshealth .org/teen/infections/skin_rashes/smallpox.html#

5. Centers for Disease Control and Prevention. (2004, December 30). Smallpox disease overview. Retrieved from www.bt.cdc.gov/agent/smallpox/overview/disease -facts.asp

6. Ibid.

7. World Health Organization. (2011, May 21). Smallpox. Retrieved from www .who.int/mediacentre/factsheets/smallpox/en/

8. D. R. Hopkins. (1983). *Princes and peasants: Smallpox in history*. Chicago: University of Chicago Press.

9. A. S. Lyons & R. J. Petrucelli. (1987). *Medicine: An illustrated history*. New York: Abradale Press.

10. K. Carr. (2011, October 21). Smallpox. Retrieved from www.historyforkids .org/learn/science/medicine/smallpox.htm

11. World Health Organization. (2011, May 21).

12. N. Barquet & P. Domingo. (1997). Smallpox: The triumph over the most terrible of the ministers of death. *Annals of Internal Medicine, 127*(8:1), 635–642.

13. H. Markel. (2011, February 28). Life, liberty and the pursuit of vaccines. *New York Times*. Retrieved from www.nytimes.com

14. D. Perlin & A. Cohen. (2002). *The complete idiot's guide to dangerous diseases and epidemics*. New York: Alpha Books.

15. Anonymous. (2011, August 25). Hemoglobin: Magical colors of the power red. Stanford School of Medicine Blood Center. Retrieved from http://bloodcenter .stanford.edu/blog/archives/2011/08/magical-powers.html

16. N. R. Finsen. (1895). The red light treatment of small-pox. *British Medical Journal, 2*(1823), 1412–1414.

17. U.S. National Library of Medicine. (2011, December 9). Smallpox: A great and terrible scourge. Retrieved from www.nlm.nih.gov/exhibition/smallpox/ sp_threat.html

18. Ibid.

19. Ibid.

20. P. Halsall. (Ed.). (1998, July). Modern history sourcebook: Lady Mary Wortley Montagu (1689–1762): Smallpox vaccination in Turkey. Fordham University Internet History Sourcebooks Project. Retrieved from www.fordham.edu/halsall/ mod/montagu-smallpox.asp

21. B. Montague. (2006, February 22). Lady Mary Wortley Montagu, 1689–1762. The Montague Millennium. Retrieved from www.montaguemillennium.com/ familyresearch/h_1762_mary.htm

22. C. Case & K. Chung. (1997). Montagu and Jenner: The campaign against smallpox. *SIM News, 47*(2), 58–60.

23. R. Mestel. (2002, December 15). Smallpox ravaged world for eons. *Los Angeles Times.* Retrieved from http://articles.latimes.com/2002/dec/15/science/sci-pox history15/2

24. S. Riedel. (2005). Edward Jenner and the history of smallpox and vaccination. *Baylor University Medical Center Proceedings, 18*(1), 21–25.

25. Ibid.

26. Ibid.

CHAPTER 3

1. Centers for Disease Control and Prevention. (2003). History and epidemiology of global smallpox eradication. [PowerPoint slides]. Retrieved from www.bt.cdc.gov/ agent/smallpox/training/overview/pdf/eradicationhistory.pdf

2. Ibid.

3. C. E. Johnson, J. Whitwell, M. L. Kumar, D. R. Nalin, L. W. Chui, & R. G. Marusyk. (1994). Measles vaccine immunogenicity in 6-versus 15-month-old infants born to mothers in the measles vaccine era. *Pediatrics, 93*(6), 939–942.

4. Advisory Committee on Immunization Practices. (1998). Measles, mumps and rubella—vaccine use and strategies for elimination of measles, rubella and congenital rubella syndrome and control of mumps: Recommendation of the advisory committee on immunization practices. *Morbidity and Mortality Weekly, 47*(RR-8), 1–57.

CHAPTER 4

1. B. Madea, F. Mußhoff, & G. Berghaus. (2006). *Verkehrsmedizin. Fahreignung, Fahrsicherheit, Unfallrekonstruktion.* Köln: Deutscher Ärzte-Verlag.

2. U.S. Department of Health and Human Services. (2008, September). Aluminum CAS # 7429-90-5. Agency for Toxic Substances and Disease Registry. Division of Toxicology and Environmental Medicine. Retrieved from www.atsdr.cdc.gov/tfacts22.pdf

3. Vaccine Education Center at the Children's Hospital of Philadelphia. (2009, Spring). Aluminum in vaccines: What you should know. Retrieved from www.chop.edu/export/download/pdfs/articles/vaccine-education-center/aluminum.pdf

4. Ibid.

5. Ibid.

6. P. Offit & R. Jew. (2003). Addressing parents' concerns: Do vaccines contain harmful preservatives, adjuvants, additives or residuals? *Pediatrics, 112*(6), 1394–1397.

7. Institute for Vaccine Safety. (2011, October 10). Components of DTaP, hep B and IPV vaccine. Johns Hopkins Bloomberg School of Public Health. Retrieved from www.vaccinesafety.edu/components-DTaP-HepB-IPV.htm

8. Vaccine Education Center at the Children's Hospital of Philadelphia. (2011, October). Hot topics: Aluminum. Retrieved from www.chop.edu/service/vaccine-education-center/hot-topics/aluminum.html

9. L. Markowitz, E. Dunne, M. Saraiya, L. Hershel, C. Harrell, & E. Unger. (2007). Quadrivalent human papillomavirus vaccine. *Morbidity and Mortality Weekly, 56*(RR02), 1–24.

10. T. Jefferson, M. Rudin, & C. DiPietrantonj. (2004). Adverse events after immunisation with aluminium-containing DTP vaccines: Systematic review of the evidence. *The Lancet Infectious Diseases, 4*(2), 84–90.

11. Center for Food Safety. (2009, May 1). Risk in brief: Formaldehyde in food. The Government of the Hong Kong Special Administrative Region. Retrieved from www.cfs.gov.hk/english/programme/programme_rafs/programme_rafs_fa_02_09.html

12. Institute for Vaccine Safety. (2011, October 3). Components of DTaP vaccine. Johns Hopkins Bloomberg School of Public Health. Retrieved from www.vaccinesafety.edu/components-DTaP.htm

13. Center for Food Safety. (2009, May 1).

14. Centers for Disease Control and Prevention. (2011). Vaccine excipient and media summary. In W. Atkinson, S. Wolfe, & J. Hamborsky (Eds.), *Epidemiology and prevention of vaccine-preventable diseases* (12th ed.). Washington DC: Public Health Foundation. Retrieved from www.cdc.gov/vaccines/pubs/pinkbook/downloads/appendices/B/excipient-table-1.pdf

15. Institute for Vaccine Safety. (2011, October 3). Components of DTaP vaccine.

16. Institute for Vaccine Safety. (2011, October 10). Components of DTaP, hep B and IPV vaccine.

17. Centers for Disease Control and Prevention. (2011). Vaccine excipient and media summary.

18. Ibid.

19. Ibid.

20. Institute for Vaccine Safety. (2011, October 3). Components of seasonal influenza vaccines. Johns Hopkins Bloomberg School of Public Health. Retrieved from www.vaccinesafety.edu/components-Influenza.htm

21. Food Standards Australia New Zealand. (2003, June). Sodium glutamate: A safety assessment. Retrieved from www.foodstandards.gov.au/_srcfiles/MSG%20 Technical%20Report.pdf

22. Ibid.

23. Ibid.

24. WebMD. (2004, December 8). RxList: Neomycin sulfate indications and dosage. Retrieved from www.rxlist.com/neomycin_sulfate-drug.htm

25. Centers for Disease Control and Prevention. (2011). Vaccine excipient and media summary.

26. Ibid.

27. Ibid.

28. Ibid.

29. Institute for Vaccine Safety. (2011, October 3). Components of DTaP vaccine. Johns Hopkins Bloomberg School of Public Health. Retrieved from www.vaccine safety.edu/components-DTaP.htm

30. Centers for Disease Control and Prevention. (2011). Vaccine excipient and media summary.

31. Institute for Vaccine Safety. (2011, October 10). Components of DTaP, hep B and IPV vaccine. Johns Hopkins Bloomberg School of Public Health. Retrieved from www.vaccinesafety.edu/components-DTaP-HepBIPV.htm

32. Institute for Vaccine Safety. (2011, June 13). Components of vaccines. Johns Hopkins Bloomberg School of Public Health. Retrieved from www.vaccinesafety .edu/components.htm

33. Ibid.

34. Ibid.

35. Ibid.

36. Ibid.

37. Ibid.

38. Institute for Vaccine Safety. (2011, October 3). Components of MMR vaccines. Johns Hopkins Bloomberg School of Public Health. Retrieved from www .vaccinesafety.edu/components-MMR.htm

39. Ibid.

40. Ibid.

41. Hostess Brands, Inc. (n.d.). Wonder Smartwhite bread. Retrieved from www .wonderbread.com/white-bread.html

42. Ibid.

43. Bumble Bee Foods, LLC. (n.d.). Current topics. Retrieved from www .bumblebee.com/faqs

44. Ibid.

45. Institute for Vaccine Safety. (2011, June 13). Components of vaccines.

46. Environmental Working Group. (n.d.). 2011 shopper's guide to pesticides in produce. Retrieved from www.ewg.org/foodnews/

47. Pontifical Academy for Life. (2005, July 26). Vatican official clarifies stance on vaccines from fetal tissue. Retrieved from www.lifesitenews.com/news/archive/ldn/1950/72/5072604

48. K. Nelson & M. Bauman. (2003). Thimerosal and autism. *Pediatrics, 111*(3), 674–679.

49. Ibid.

50. M. E. Pichichero et al. (2008). Mercury levels in newborns and infants after receipt of thimerosal-containing vaccines. *Pediatrics, 121*(2), 208–214.

51. Ibid.

CHAPTER 5

1. C. S. Demirci & W. Abuhammour. (2011, November 23). Pediatric diphtheria. Medscape: Drugs, diseases and procedures. Retrieved from http://emedicine.medscape.com/article/963334-overview

2. Ibid.

3. D. Cherry. (1999). Pertussis in the pre-antibiotic and pre-vaccine era with an emphasis on adult pertussis. *Clinical Infectious Diseases, 28,* S107–111.

4. Ibid.

5. J. Flanders. (2005). *Inside the Victorian home: A portrait of domestic life in Victorian England* (p. 77). New York: Norton.

6. J. Miller. (1998). *Becoming Laura Ingalls Wilder: The woman behind the legend.* Columbia: University of Missouri Press.

7. M. Davis, M. Patel, & A. Gebremariam. (2004). Decline in varicella-related hospitalizations and expenditures for children and adults after introduction of varicella vaccine in the United States. *Pediatrics, 114*(3), 786–792.

8. Ibid.

9. K. Todar. (n.d.). Diphtheria. *Todar's online textbook of biology.* Retrieved from www.textbookofbacteriology.net/diphtheria.html

10. Ibid.

11. Ibid.

12. Ibid.

13. Ibid.

14. Ibid.

15. Ibid.

16. Ibid.

17. Centers for Disease Control and Prevention. (2011, June 24). What would happen if we stopped vaccinations? Retrieved from www.cdc.gov/vaccines/vac-gen/whatifstop.htm

18. Ibid.

19. Ibid.
20. World Health Organization. (2006). WHO position paper on haemophilus influenzae type b conjugate vaccines. *Weekly Epidemiology Record, 81*(47), 445–452.
21. Immunization Action Coalition. (2011, March). Hib disease: Questions and answers. Retrieved from www.vaccineinformation.org/hib/qandadis.asp
22. Ibid.
23. Ibid.
24. M. Rathore & A. Mirza. (2010, July 8). Pediatric haemophilus influenzae infection. Retrieved from http://emedicine.medscape.com/article/964317 -overview#showall
25. Ibid.
26. Immunization Action Coalition. (2011, March). Hib disease: Questions and answers.
27. Centers for Disease Control and Prevention. (2011, November 27). Genital HPV infection—fact sheet. Retrieved from www.cdc.gov/std/hpv/stdfact-hpv.htm
28. National Cancer Institute. (2011, September 9). Human papillomavirus (HPV) vaccines. Retrieved from www.cancer.gov/cancertopics/factsheet/prevention/ HPV-vaccine
29. Hepatitis B Foundation. (2009, October 21). About hepatitis B: Statistics. Retrieved from www.hepb.org/hepb/statistics.htm
30. Ibid.
31. Ibid.
32. World Health Organization. (2008, August). Hepatitis B fact sheet. Retrieved from www.who.int/mediacentre/factsheets/fs204/en/
33. Ibid.
34. National Network for Immunization Information. (2008, March 3). Why is hepatitis B vaccination recommended for all infants, children, and adolescents? Retrieved from www.immunizationinfo.org/issues/general/why-hepatitis-b-immuni zation-recommended-all-infants-children-and-adolescents
35. R. Knox. (2005, October 5). 1918 killer flu reconstructed. National Public Radio. Retrieved from www.npr.org/templates/story/story.php?storyId=4946718
36. S. Reinberg. (2011, August 9). CDC urges all Americans to get flu shots. *USA Today.* Retrieved from http://yourlife.usatoday.com/
37. L. M. Ellman et al. (2010). Structural brain alterations in schizophrenia following fetal exposure to the inflammatory cytokine interleukin-8. *Schizophrenia Research, 121*(1–3), 46–54.
38. A. A. Eick et al. (2011). Maternal influenza vaccination and effect on influenza virus infection in young infants. *Archives of Pediatric and Adolescent Medicine, 165*(2), 104–111. doi:10.1001/archpediatrics.2010.192
39. M. Greger. (2006). *Bird flu: A virus of our own hatching.* Brooklyn, NY: Lantern Books. Retrieved from http://birdflubook.com/a.php?id=40
40. Centers for Disease Control and Prevention. (2009, August 31). Complications of measles. Retrieved from www.cdc.gov/measles/about/complications.html
41. Ibid.

42. Centers for Disease Control and Prevention. (2011, June 29). Measles: Make sure your child is fully immunized. Retrieved from www.cdc.gov/features/measles/

43. Centers for Disease Control and Prevention. (2011, May 27). Measles—United States, January–May 20, 2011. *Morbidity and Mortality Weekly, 60*(20), 666–668.

44. New York State Department of Health. (2010, October). Mumps. Retrieved from www.health.ny.gov/diseases/communicable/mumps/fact_sheet.htm

45. Ibid.

46. National Network for Immunization Information. (2008, December 16). Pertussis (whooping cough): Understanding the disease. Retrieved from www .immunizationinfo.org/vaccines/pertussis-whooping-cough

47. J. Klein. (2010, September). Polio. *Kids Health*. Retrieved from http:// kidshealth.org/parent/infections/bacterial_viral/polio.html#

48. Ibid.

49. A. T. Curns, C. A. Steiner, M. Barrett, K. Hunter, E. Wilson, & U. D. Parashar. (2010). Reduction in acute gastroenteritis hospitalizations among US children after introduction of rotavirus vaccine: Analysis of hospital discharge data from 18 states. *Journal of Infectious Diseases, 201*, 1617–1624.

50. Centers for Disease Control and Prevention (2012, January 25). Vaccine recommendations for infants and children. Retrieved from wwwnc.cdc.gov/travel/yellow book/2012/chapter-7-international-travel-infants-children/vaccine-recommendations -for-infants-and-children.htm

51. M. Hunt. (2011, May 24). Rubella (German measles) virus. Microbiology and Immunology On-line. University of South Carolina School of Medicine. Retrieved from http://pathmicro.med.sc.edu/mhunt/rubella.htm
Ibid.

52. Centers for Disease Control and Prevention. (1990). Current trends tetanus— United States, 1987 and 1988. *Morbidity and Mortality Weekly, 39*(3), 37–41.

53. B. Pascual, E. McGinley, L. Zanardi, M. Cortese, & T. Murphy. (2003). Tetanus surveillance 1998–2000. *Morbidity and Mortality Weekly, 52*(SS03), 1–8.

CHAPTER 6

1. M. Smith & C. Woods. (2010). On-time vaccine receipt in the first year does not adversely affect neuropsychological outcomes. *Pediatrics, 125*(6), 1134–1141.

2. Harvard Center for Risk Analysis. (2009). Causes of death. Harvard School of Public Health. Retrieved from www.hcra.harvard.edu/quiz.html

3. T. Tran. (2009). Management of hepatitis B in pregnancy: Weighing the options. *Cleveland Clinic Journal of Medicine, 76*, 525–529.

4. National Network for Immunization Information. (2009, July 16). Varicella: Understanding the disease. Retrieved from www.immunizationinfo.org/vaccines/ varicella-chickenpox

5. Centers for Disease Control and Prevention. (2011, April 21). Possible side-effects from vaccines. Retrieved from www.cdc.gov/vaccines/vac-gen/side-effects.htm

6. World Health Organization. (2011, September 23). Diphtheria reported cases. Retrieved from http://apps.who.int/immunization_monitoring/en/globalsummary/timeseries/tsincidencedip.htm

7. Centers for Disease Control and Prevention. (2011, April 21). Possible side-effects from vaccines.

8. Centers for Disease Control and Prevention. (2011, August 4). Hepatitis A FAQs for health officials. Retrieved from www.cdc.gov/hepatitis/HAV/HAVfaq.htm

9. American Academy of Pediatrics. (n.d.). Why immunize? Retrieved from www2.aap.org/immunization/families/whyimmunize.html

10. Centers for Disease Control and Prevention. (2011, April 21). Possible side-effects from vaccines.

11. Ibid.

12. J. Heilprin. (2011, April 21). Measles outbreak in Europe, especially France. *Huffington Post.* Retrieved from www.huffingtonpost.com/2011/04/21/europe-measles-outbreak-france_n_851911.html

13. Centers for Disease Control and Prevention. (2011, April 21). Possible side-effects from vaccines.

14. Centers for Disease Control and Prevention. (2011, March 11). Meningitis: Questions and answers. Retrieved from www.cdc.gov/meningitis/about/faq.html

15. M. C. Thigpen et al. (2011). Bacterial meningitis in the United States 1998–2007. *New England Journal of Medicine, 364*(21), 2016–2025.

16. Centers for Disease Control and Prevention. (2010, February 12). Update: Mumps outbreak New York and New Jersey, June 2009–January 2010. *Morbidity and Mortality Weekly Report, 59*(5), 125–129.

17. Centers for Disease Control and Prevention. (2011, April 21). Possible side-effects from vaccines.

18. V. R. Racaniello. (2006). One hundred years of poliovirus pathogenesis. *Virology, 344*(1), 9–16. doi:10.1016/j.virol.2005.09.015

19. Ibid.

20. Centers for Disease Control and Prevention. (2011, December 1). Pneumonia can be prevented: Vaccines can help. Retrieved from www.cdc.gov/Features/Pneumonia/

21. Ibid.

22. J. Klein. (2009, September). Rotavirus. Retrieved from http://kidshealth.org/parent/infections/stomach/rotavirus.html#

23. Ibid.

24. Centers for Disease Control and Prevention. (2011, April 21). Possible side-effects from vaccines.

25. D. Dire. (2011, September 20). Tetanus in emergency medicine. Retrieved from http://emedicine.medscape.com/article/786414-overview#a0199

26. J. Steckelberg. (2010, December 16). What happens if you get tetanus shots too close together—within a few years instead of the recommended 10 years? Retrieved from www.mayoclinic.com/health/tetanus-shots/AN01497

27. Centers for Disease Control and Prevention. (2011, August 22). Pertussis (whooping cough) outbreaks. Retrieved from www.cdc.gov/pertussis/outbreaks.html

28. Centers for Disease Control and Prevention. (2011, April 21). Possible side-effects from vaccines.

29. M. J. Goodman & J. Nordin. (2006). Vaccine Adverse Event Reporting System reporting source: A possible source of bias in longitudinal studies. *Pediatrics,* *117*(2), 387–390.

30. Centers for Disease Control and Prevention. (2011, October 27). Human papillomavirus (HPV). Retrieved from www.cdc.gov/hpv/

CHAPTER 7

1. A. J. Wakefield et al. (1998). Ileal-lymphoid-nodular hyperplasia, non-specific colitis, and pervasive developmental disorder in children. *The Lancet* (9103), *351,* 637–641.

2. Anonymous. (2010). Retraction: Ileal-lymphoid-nodular hyperplasia, non-specific colitis, and pervasive developmental disorder in children. *The Lancet,* *375*(9713), 445.

3. M. Booth. (2011, November 29). Colorado parents rank second in nation for vaccine refusals. *Denver Post.* Retrieved from www.denverpost.com

4. Wakefield et al. (1998). 641.

5. Ibid.

6. B. Deer. (2011, August 4). Royal Free facilitates attack on MMR in medical school single shots videotape. Retrieved from http://briandeer.com/wakefield/royal -video.htm

7. R. M. Anderson & R. M. May. (1985). Vaccination and herd immunity to infectious diseases. *Nature, 318,* 323–329.

8. A. Ekbom, P. Daszak, W. Kraaz, & A. J. Wakefield. (1996). Crohn's disease after in-utero measles virus exposure. *The Lancet, 348*(9026), 515–517.

9. American Academy of Pediatrics. (2011, January 20). What parents should know about measles-mumps-rubella (MMR) vaccine and autism. Retrieved from www2.aap.org/immunization/families/autismfacts.html

10. B. Deer. (2011, July 22). Revealed: Wakefield's secret first MMR patent claims "safer measles vaccine." Retrieved from http://briandeer.com/wakefield/ vaccine-patent.htm

11. A. J. Wakefield & H. Fundenberg. (1998, April 6). U.K. patent application GB 2 325 856 A. Retrieved from http://briandeer.com/mmr/1998-vaccine-patent.pdf

12. S. Barrett & R. S. Baratz. (2005, April 20). Disciplinary actions against Herman Hugh Fudenberg, M.D. Retrieved from www.casewatch.org/board/med/ fudenberg/1995order.shtml

13. B. Deer. (2011, August 5). Royal Free autism pill partner, Herman Hugh Fudenberg, wasn't fit to prescribe. Retrieved from http://briandeer.com/wakefield/ hugh-fudenberg.htm

14. B. Deer. (2011b). How the vaccine crisis was meant to make money. *British Medical Journal, 342*(7789), 136–142. doi:10.1136/bmj.c5258

15. R. Verreault, D. Laurin, J. Lindsay, & G. De Serres. (2001). Past exposure to vaccines and subsequent risk of Alzheimer's disease. *Canadian Medical Association Journal, 165*(11), 1495–1498.

16. B. Deer. (2006, December 31). MMR scare doctor got legal aid fortune. *Sunday Times* (London). Record number 908788052.

17. S. H. Murch et al. (2004). Retraction of an interpretation. *The Lancet, 363*(9411), 750.

18. B. Deer. (2011a). How the case against the MMR vaccine was fixed. *British Medical Journal, 342*, 77–82. doi:10.1136/bmj.c5347

19. T. Carter. (2004, November 18). *MMR: What they didn't tell you.* London: Channel 4.

20. General Medical Council. (2010, May 24). Determination on serious professional misconduct (SPM) and sanction. Retrieved from www.gmc-uk.org/Wakefield_SPM_and_SANCTION.pdf_32595267.pdf

21. S. Dominus. (2011, April 24). The crash and burn of an autism guru. *New York Times.* Retrieved from www.nytimes.com

CHAPTER 8

1. K. M. Madsen et al. (2003). Thimerosal and the occurrence of autism: Negative ecological evidence from Danish population-based data. *Pediatrics, 112*, 604–606. doi:10.1542/peds.112.3.204

2. N. Andrews, E. Miller, A. Grant, J. Stowe, V. Osborn, & B. Taylor. (2004). Thimerosal exposure in infants and developmental disorders: A retrospective cohort study in the United Kingdom does not support a causal association. *Pediatrics, 114*, 584–591. doi:10.1542/peds.2003-1177-L

3. S. K. Parker, B. Schwartz, J. Todd, & L. K. Pickering. (2004). Thimerosal-containing vaccines and autistic spectrum disorder: A critical review of published original data. *Pediatrics, 114*, 793–804.

4. M. E. Pichichero et al. (2008). Mercury levels in newborns and infants after receipt of thimerosal-containing vaccines. *Pediatrics, 121*(2), 208–214.

5. E. Fombonne, R. Zakarian, A. Bennett, L. Meng, & D. McLean-Heywood. (2006). Pervasive developmental disorders in Montreal, Quebec, Canada: Prevalence and links with immunizations. *Pediatrics, 118*(1), E139–E150. doi:10.1542/peds.2005-2993

6. H. Peltola, A. Patja, P. Leinikki, M. Valle, I. Davidkin, & M. Paunio. (1998). No evidence for measles, mumps, and rubella vaccine-associated inflammatory bowel disease or autism in a 14-year prospective study. *The Lancet, 351*(9112), 1327.

7. B. Taylor et al. (1999). Autism and measles, mumps, and rubella vaccine: No epidemiological evidence for a causal association. *The Lancet, 353*(9169), 2026–2029.

8. K. M. Madsen et al. (2002). A population-based study of measles, mumps, and rubella vaccination and autism. *New England Journal of Medicine, 347*(19), 1477–1482.

9. M. Hornig et al. (2008). Lack of association between measles virus vaccine and autism with enteropathy: A case-control study. *PLoS One, 3*(9), E3140. doi:10.1371/journal.pone.0003140

10. T. Uchiyama, M. Kurosawa, & Y. Inaba. (2007). MMR-vaccine and regression in autism spectrum disorders: Negative results presented from Japan. *Journal of Autism and Developmental Disorders, 37*(2), 210–217.

11. I. Hertz-Picciotto, P. Green, L. Delwiche, R. Hansen, C. Walker, & I. Pessah. (2010). Blood mercury concentrations in CHARGE Study children with and without autism. *Environmental Health Perspectives, 118*(1), 161–166. doi:10.1289/ehp.0900736

12. A. Asif Doja & W. Roberts. (2006). Immunizations and autism: A review of the literature. *Canadian Journal of Neurological Sciences, 33*(4), 341–346.

13. A. Makela, J. Nuorti, & H. Peltola. (2002). Neurologic disorders after measles-mumps-rubella vaccination. *Pediatrics, 110*(5), 957–963.

14. M. W. State. (2010). The genetics of child psychiatric disorders: Focus on autism and Tourette syndrome. *Neuron, 68*(2), 254–269. doi:10.1016/j.neuron.2010.10.004

15. P. Szatmari et al. (2007). Mapping autism risk loci using genetic linkage and chromosomal rearrangements. *Nature Genetics, 39*(3), 319–328.

16. D. Arking et al. (2008). Association between microdeletion and microduplication at 16p11.2 and autism. *New England Journal of Medicine, 358*(7), 667–675.

17. R. Muhle, S. V. Trentacoste, & I. Rapin. (2004). The genetics of autism. *Pediatrics, 113*(5), E472–E486.

18. K. Cheslack-Postava, K. Liu, & P. S. Bearman. (2011). Closely spaced pregnancies are associated with increased odds of autism in California sibling births. *Pediatrics, 127*(2), 246–253.

19. J. F. Shelton, D. J. Tancredi, & I. Hertz-Picciotto. (2010). Independent and dependent contributions of advanced maternal and paternal ages to autism risk. *Autism Research, 3*, 30–39.

20. J. Daniels et al. (2008). Parental psychiatric disorders associated with autism spectrum disorders in the offspring. *Pediatrics, 121*(5), E1357.

21. H. Atladóttir et al. (2010). Maternal infection requiring hospitalization during pregnancy and autism spectrum disorders. *Journal of Autism and Developmental Disorders, 40*(12), 1423–1430.

22. E. Courchesne et al. (2011). Neuron number and size in prefrontal cortex of children with autism. *Journal of the American Medical Association, 306*(18), 2001–2010.

23. C. J. Limperopoulos. (2008). Positive screening for autism in ex-preterm infants: Prevalence and risk factors. *Pediatrics, 121*(4), 758.

24. C. J. Limperopoulos. (2007). Does cerebral injury in premature infants contribute to the high prevalence of long-term cognitive, learning, and behavioral disability in survivors? *Pediatrics, 120*(3), 584.

25. C. M. Schumann et al. (2004). The amygdala is enlarged in children but not adolescents with autism; the hippocampus is enlarged at all ages. *Journal of Neuroscience, 24*(28), 6392–6401. doi:10.1523/JNEUROSCI.1297-04.2004

26. A. Kolevzon, R. Gross, & A. Reichenberg. (2007). Prenatal and perinatal risk factors for autism. *Archives of Pediatric and Adolescent Medicine, 161,* 326–333.

27. N. Yirmiya & T. Charman. (2010). The prodrome of autism: Early behavioral and biological signs, regression, peri- and post-natal development and genetics. *Journal of Child Psychology and Psychiatry, 51*(4), 432–458. doi:10.1111/j.1469-7610.2010.02214.x

28. American Psychiatric Association. (2000). Autism. *Diagnostic and statistical manual of mental disorders: DSM-IV-TR* (4th ed.). Washington, DC: American Psychiatric Association.

29. B. Siegel, C. Pliner, J. Eschler, & G. R. Elliot. (1988). How children with autism are diagnosed: Difficulties in identification of children with multiple developmental delays. *Developmental and Behavioral Pediatrics, 9*(4), 199–204.

30. J. Osterling & G. Dawson. (1994). Early recognition of children with autism: A study of first birthday home videotapes. *Journal of Autism and Developmental Disorders, 24*(3), 247–257.

31. M. Yeargin-Allsopp, C. Rice, R. Karapurkar, N. Doernberg, C. Boyle, & C. Murphy. (2003). Prevalence of autism in a US metropolitan area. *Journal of the American Medical Association, 289*(1), 49–55.

32. M. S. Gernsbacher, M. Dawson, & H. H. Goldsmith. (2005). Three reasons not to believe in an autism epidemic. *Current Directions in Psychological Science, 14,* 55–58. doi:10.1111/j.0963-7214.2005.00334

CHAPTER 9

1. M. R. Geier & D. A. Geier. (2005). The potential importance of steroids in the treatment of autistic spectrum disorders and other disorders involving mercury toxicity. *Medical Hypotheses, 64*(5), 946–954. doi:10.1016/j.mehy.2004.11.018

2. S. Bernard, A. Enayati, L. Redwood, H. Roger, & T. Binstock. (2001). Autism: A novel form of mercury poisoning. *Medical Hypotheses, 56*(4), 462–471. doi:10.1054/mehy.2000.1281

3. S. Barrett. (2003, October 9). Dr. Mark Geier severely criticized. Retrieved from www.casewatch.org/civil/geier.shtml

4. U.S. Department of Health and Human Services. (n.d.). About the VAERS program. Retrieved from http://vaers.hhs.gov/about/index

5. Centers for Disease Control and Prevention. (1999). Withdrawal of rotavirus vaccine recommendation. *Morbidity and Mortality Weekly, 48*(43), 1007.

6. J. R. Laidler. (2005, July 27). Chelation and autism. *Neurodiversity Weblog.* Retrieved from http://neurodiversity.com/weblog/article/14/chelation-autism

7. Ibid.

8. M. J. Goodman & J. Nordin. (2006). Vaccine Adverse Event Reporting System reporting source: A possible source of bias in longitudinal studies. *Pediatrics, 117*(2), 387–390. doi:10.1542/peds.2004-2687

9. P. A. Offit. (2008). *Autism's false prophets: Bad science, risky medicine, and the search for a cure.* New York: Columbia University Press.

10. U.S. Department of Health and Human Services. (n.d.). VAERS data. Retrieved from http://vaers.hhs.gov/data/index

11. D. A. Geier & M. R. Geier. (2002). Serious neurological conditions following pertussis immunization: An analysis of endotoxin levels, the Vaccine Adverse Events Reporting System (VAERS) database and literature review. *Pediatric Rehabilitation, 5*(3), 177–182. doi:10.1080/1363849021000054031

12. D. A. Geier & M. R. Geier. (2003). An assessment of the impact of thimerosal on childhood neurodevelopmental disorders. *Pediatric Rehabilitation, 6*(2), 97. doi:10.1080/1363849031000139315

13. D. A. Geier & M. R. Geier. (2004b). Neurodevelopmental disorders following thimerosal-containing childhood immunizations: A follow-up analysis. *International Journal of Toxicology, 23*(6), 369–376. doi:10.1080/10915810490902038

14. D. A. Geier & M. R. Geier. (2006). An evaluation of the effects of thimerosal on neurodevelopmental disorders reported following DTP and Hib vaccines in comparison to DTPH vaccine in the United States. *Journal of Toxicology and Environmental Health: Part A, 69*(15), 1481–1495. doi:10.1080/15287390500364556

15. M. R. Geier, D. A. Geier, & A. C. Zahalsky. (2003). Influenza vaccination and Guillain Barre syndrome. *Clinical Immunology, 107*(2), 116. doi:10.1016/S1521-6616(03)00046-9

16. D. A. Geier & M. R. Geier. (2005). A case-control study of serious autoimmune adverse events following hepatitis B immunization. *Autoimmunity, 38*(4), 295–301. doi:10.1080/08916930500144484

17. D. A. Geier & M. R. Geier. (2004a). An evaluation of serious neurological disorders following immunization: A comparison of whole-cell pertussis and acellular pertussis vaccines. *Brain and Development, 26*(5), 296–300. doi:10.1016/S0387-7604(03)00169-4

18. WebMD. (2009, June 30). Chelation therapy: Topic overview. Retrieved from www.webmd.com/balance/tc/chelation-therapy-topic-overview

19. R. A. Beauchamp et al. (2006). Deaths associated with hypocalcemia from chelation therapy: Texas, Pennsylvania, and Oregon, 2003–2005. *Journal of the American Medical Association, 295*(18), 2131–2133.

20. Laidler. (2005, July 27).

21. M. Miika. (2008). Chelation therapy trials halted. *Journal of the American Medical Association, 300*(19), 2236.

22. Research Autism. (2011, July 11). Chelation and autism. Retrieved from www.researchautism.net/autism_treatments_therapies_intervention.ikml?ra=25

23. A. J. Baxter & E. P. Krenzelok. (2008). Pediatric fatality secondary to EDTA chelation. *Clinical Toxicology, 46*, 1083–1084. doi:10.1080/15563650701261488

24. M. R. Geier & D. A. Geier. (2005).

25. Prometheus. (2006, March 12). Armchair science vs. real science. [Weblog]. Retrieved from http://photoninthedarkness.blogspot.com/2006/03/armchair-science -vs-real-science.html

26. P. B. Kaplowitz, P. W. Speiser, M. L. Windle, L. L. Levitsky, M. P. M. Poth, & S. Kemp. (2010, March 29). Precocious puberty. Retrieved from http://emedicine .medscape.com/article/924002-overview

27. Mayo Clinic. (2011, February 3). Precocious puberty: Treatment and drugs. Retrieved from www.mayoclinic.com/health/precocious-puberty/DS00883/ DSECTION=treatments-and-drugs

28. E. J. Willingham. (2011, May 5). Autism, Lupron, the Geiers, and what can science do about emotions? *Science, Society, and You.* [Weblog]. Retrieved from http:// biologyfiles.fieldofscience.com/2011/05/autism-lupron-geiers-and-what-can.html

29. B. J. Martin. (2008, October 30). TAP's patent application to give Lupron to autistic children. *Pathophilia.* [Weblog]. Retrieved from http://bmartinmd.com/2008/10/ taps-patent-application-to-giv.html

30. Ibid.

31. F. D. Royland. (2011, May 20). O'Malley ousts David Geier from autism commission. *Baltimore Sun.* Retrieved from www.baltimoresun.com

32. M. Cohn. (2011, May 19). Son of autism doctor charged with practicing without a license. *Baltimore Sun.* Retrieved from www.baltimoresun.com

33. Maryland State Board of Physicians. (2011, May 16). *Charges under the Maryland Medical Practices Act, case numbers 2008-0022 and 2009-0318.* Retrieved from www.mbp.state.md.us/BPQAPP/orders/GeierCharge05162011.pdf

34. U.S. Food and Drug Administration. (2009, March 3). Institutional review boards frequently asked questions—information sheet. Retrieved from www.fda.gov/ RegulatoryInformation/Guidances/ucm126420.htm

35. K. Siedel. (2006, June 20). An elusive institute [Weblog]. Retrieved from http://neurodiversity.com/weblog/article/98/an-elusive-institute-significant-misrep resentations-mark-geier-david-geier-the-evolution-of-the-lupron-protocol-part-two

CHAPTER 10

1. K. Stratton, A. Gable, & M. C. McCormick. (Eds.). (2001). Immunization safety review: Thimerosal-containing vaccines and neurodevelopmental disorders. Washington, DC: National Academy Press.

2. N. Andrews, E. Miller, A. Grant, J. Stowe, V. Osborn, & B. Taylor. (2004). Thimerosal exposure in infants and developmental disorders: A retrospective cohort study in the United Kingdom does not support a causal association. *Pediatrics, 114,* 584–591. doi:10.1542/peds.2003-1177-L

3. J. Heron & J. Golden. (2004). Thimerosal exposure in infants and developmental disorders: A prospective cohort study in the United Kingdom does not support a causal association. *Pediatrics, 114*(3), 577.

4. W. W. Thompson et al. (2007). Early thimerosal exposure and neuropsychological outcomes at 7 to 10 years. *New England Journal of Medicine, 357*(13), 1281–1292.

5. E. H. Cook Jr. (1999). Genetics of attention-deficit hyperactivity disorder. *Mental Retardation and Developmental Disabilities Research Reviews, 5*(3), 191–198.

6. M. Bornovalova, B. Hicks, W. Iacono, & M. McGue. (2010). Familial transmission and heritability of childhood disruptive disorders. *American Journal of Psychiatry, 167*(9), 1066–1074.

7. Ibid.

8. T. Banaschewski, K. Becker, S. Scherag, B. Franke, & D. Coghill. (2010). Molecular genetics of attention-deficit/hyperactivity disorder: An overview. *European Child and Adolescent Psychiatry, 19*(3), 237–257. doi:10.1007/s00787-010-0090-z

9. H. Courvoisie, S. R. Hooper, C. Fine, L. Kwock, & M. Castillo. (2004). Neurometabolic functioning and neuropsychological correlates in children with ADHD-H: Preliminary findings. *Journal of Neuropsychiatry and Clinical Neurosciences, 16,* 63–69.

10. B. Kim, J. Lee, M. Shin, S. Cho, & D. Lee. (2002). Regional cerebral perfusion abnormalities in attention deficit/hyperactivity disorder: Statistical parametric mapping analysis. *European Archives of Psychiatry and Clinical Neuroscience, 252*(5), 219.

11. J. V. Chandan, S. A. Bunge, N. M. Dudukovic, C. A. Zalecki, G. R. Elliot, & J. D. E. Gabrielli. (2005). Altered neural substrates of cognitive control in childhood ADHD: Evidence from functional magnetic resonance imaging. *American Journal of Psychiatry, 162*(9), 1605–1613.

12. D. J. Cox, B. P. Kovatchev, J. B. Morris, C. Phillips, R. J. Hill, & L. Merkel. (1998). Electroencephalographic and psychometric differences between boys with and without attention-deficit/hyperactivity disorder (ADHD): A pilot study. *Applied Psychophysiology and Biofeedback, 23*(3), 179–188.

13. E. R. Sowell, P. M. Thompson, S. E. Welcome, A. L. Henkenius, A. W. Toga, & B. S. Peterson. (2003). Cortical abnormalities in children and adolescents with attention-deficit hyperactivity disorder. *The Lancet, 362*(9397), 1699–1707.

14. J. Serene, M. Ashtari, P. R. Szeszko, & S. Kumra. (2007). Neuroimaging studies of children with serious emotional disturbances: A selective review. *Canadian Journal of Psychiatry, 52*(3), 135–145.

15. P. Shaw et al. (2007). Attention-deficit/hyperactivity disorder is characterized by a delay in cortical maturation. *Proceedings of the National Academy of Sciences of the United States of America, 104*(49), 19649–19654.

16. D. A. Christakis, F. J. Zimmerman, D. L. DiGiuseppe, & C. A. McCarty. (2004). Early television exposure and subsequent attentional problems in children. *Pediatrics, 113,* 708–713.

17. B. M. Kuehn. (2010). Increased risk of ADHD associated with early exposure to pesticides, PCBs. *Journal of the American Medical Association, 304*(1), 27–28.

18. A. Marks et al. (2010). Organophosphate pesticide exposure and attention in young Mexican-American children: The CHAMACOS Study. *Environmental Health Perspectives, 118*(12), 1768–1774.

19. T. Banerjee, F. Middleton, & S. V. Faraone. (2007). Environmental risk factors for attention-deficit hyperactivity disorder. *Acta Paediatrica, 96*(9), 1269–1274. doi:10.1111/j.1651-2227.2007.00430.x

20. Asthma and Allergy Foundation of America. (n.d.). Allergy facts and figures. Retrieved from www.aafa.org/display.cfm?id=9&sub=30#_ftnref1

21. L. Nilsson, N. I. M. Kjellman, & B. Bjorksten. (1998). A randomized controlled trial of the effect of pertussis vaccines on atopic disease. *Archives of Pediatrics and Adolescent Medicine, 152*(8), 734–738. Document ID: 33018374

22. Ibid.

23. T. M. McKeever, S. A. Lewis, C. Smith, & R. Hubbard. (2004). Vaccination and allergic disease: A birth cohort study. *American Journal of Public Health, 94*(6), 985–989.

24. L. Nilsson, N. I. M. Kjellman, & B. Bjorksten (2003). Allergic disease at the age of 7 years after pertussis vaccination in infancy. *Archives of Pediatric and Adolescent Medicine, 157*(12), 1184–1189.

25. McKeever et al. (2004).

26. J. S. Alm, G. Lilja, G. Pershagen, & A. Scheynius. (1997). Early BCG vaccination and development of atopy. *The Lancet, 350*(9075), 400–403.

27. Nilsson et al. (2003).

28. McKeever et al. (2004).

29. H. P. Roost et al. (2004). Influence of MMR-vaccinations and diseases on atopic sensitization and allergic symptoms in Swiss schoolchildren. *Pediatric Allergy and Immunology, 15*(5), 401–407. doi:10.1111/j.1399-3038.2004.00192.x

30. Alm et al. (1997).

31. P. A. Offit & C. J. Hackett. (2003). Addressing parents' concerns: Do vaccines cause allergic or autoimmune diseases? *Pediatrics, 111*(3), 653–660. doi:10.1542/peds.111.3.653

32. F. DeStefano et al. (2002). Childhood vaccinations and risk of asthma. *Pediatric Infectious Disease Journal, 21*, 498–504. doi:10.1097/00006454-200206000-00004

33. H. R. Anderson, J. D. Poloniecki, D. P. Strachan, R. Beasley, B. Bjorksten, & M. I. Asher. (2001). Immunization and symptoms of atopic disease in children: Results from the international study of asthma and allergies in childhood. *American Journal of Public Health, 91*(7), 1126–1129.

34. M. Bijanzadeh, P. A. Mahesh, & N. B. Ramachand. (2011). An understanding of the genetic basis of asthma. *Indian Journal of Medical Research, 134*(2), 149–161.

35. P. J. Burney, R. B. Newson, M. S. Burrows, & D. M. Wheeler. (2008). The effects of allergens in outdoor air on both atopic and nonatopic subjects with airway disease. *Allergy, 63*(5), 542–546. doi:10.1111/j.1398-9995.2007.01596.x

36. M. C. McCormack et al. (2009). In-home particle concentrations and childhood asthma morbidity. *Environmental Health Perspectives, 117*(2), 294–298.

37. K. Moore et al. (2008). Ambient ozone concentrations cause increased hospitalizations for asthma in children: An 18-year study in southern California. *Environmental Health Perspectives, 116*(8), 1063–1070.

38. D. P. Strachan. (1989). Hayfever, hygiene, and household size. *British Journal of Medicine, 299*, 1259–1269.

39. A. H. Mokdad et al. (2001). The continuing increase of diabetes in the U.S. *Diabetes Care, 24,* 412. doi:10.2337/diacare.24.2.412

40. D. C. Classen & J. B. Classen. (1997). The timing of pediatric immunization and the risk of insulin-dependent diabetes mellitus. *Infectious Diseases in Clinical Practice, 6*(7), 449–454.

41. J. B. Classen & D. C. Classen. (1999). Vertically transmitted enteroviruses and the benefits of neonatal immunization. *Diabetes Care, 22*(10), 1760–1761.

42. D. Elliman. (1999). Vaccination and type 1 diabetes mellitus: Currently no evidence of a link, but more studies are needed as vaccines change. *British Medical Journal, 318*(7192), 1159–1160.

43. A. Neu, M. Kehrer, R. Hub, & M. B. Ranke. (1997). Incidence of type 1 diabetes in Germany is not higher than predicted: Response. *Diabetes Care, 20*(11), 1799–1800.

44. T. Jefferson & V. Demicheli. (1998). No evidence that vaccines cause insulin dependent diabetes mellitus. *Journal of Epidemiology and Community Health, 52*(10), 674–675.

45. Offit & Hackett. (2003).

46. J. P. Bradfield et al. (2011). A genome-wide meta-analysis of six type 1 diabetes cohorts identifies multiple associated loci. *PLoS Genetics, 7*(9), 1–8. doi:10.1371/journal.pgen.1002293

47. P. Arora et al. (2011). Genetic polymorphisms of innate immunity-related inflammatory pathways and their association with factors related to type 2 diabetes. *BMC Medical Genetics, 12*(1), 95–103. doi:10.1186/1471-2350-12-95

48. C. Whitmore. (2010). Type 2 diabetes and obesity in adults. *British Journal of Nursing (BJN), 19*(14), 880–886.

49. L. L. Liu et al. (2010). Prevalence of overweight and obesity in youth with diabetes in USA: The SEARCH for Diabetes in Youth Study. *Pediatric Diabetes, 11*(1), 4–11. doi:10.1111/j.1399-5448.2009.00519.xx

50. B. Fletcher, M. Gulanick, & C. Lamendola. (2002). Risk factors for type 2 diabetes mellitus. *Journal of Cardiovascular Nursing, 16*(2), 17–23.

51. G. G. Soltesz, C. C. Patterson, & G. G. Dahlquist. (2007). Worldwide childhood type 1 diabetes incidence—what can we learn from epidemiology? *Pediatric Diabetes, 8*(Supp. 6), 6–14. doi:10.1111/j.1399-5448.2007.00280.x

52. M. Finucane et al. (2011). National, regional, and global trends in body-mass index since 1980: Systematic analysis of health examination surveys and epidemiological studies with 960 country-years and 9.1 million participants. *The Lancet, 377*(9765), 557–567.

53. World Health Organization. (2011, August 4). Obesity and overweight fact sheet. Retrieved from www.who.int/mediacentre/factsheets/fs311/en/

54. Mayo Clinic. (2011, May 6). Obesity: Causes. Retrieved from www.mayoclinic.com/health/obesity/DS00314/DSECTION=causes

55. American Academy of Child and Adolescent Psychiatry. (2011, March). Facts for families: Obesity in children and teens. Retrieved from www.aacap.org/galleries/FactsForFamilies/79_obesity_in_children_and_teens.pdf

56. A. A. Vasilakopoulou & C. W. le Roux. (2007). Could a virus contribute to weight gain? *International Journal of Obesity, 31*(9), 1350–1356. doi:10.1038/sj.ijo.0803623

57. R. L. Atkinson. (2007). Viruses as an etiology of obesity. *Mayo Clinic Proceedings, 82*(10), 1192–1198.

CHAPTER 11

1. National Network for Immunization Information. (n.d.). About NNii: Funding. Retrieved from www.immunizationinfo.org/about-nnii/funding

2. D. Olmstead. (n.d.). A letter from the editor. *Age of Autism.* Retrieved from www.ageofautism.com/a-welcome-from-dan-olmste.html

3. K. Doheny. (2009, May 11). Researchers see recovery from autism: Study shows some children may "move off" the autistic spectrum. WebMD Health News. Retrieved from www.webmd.com/brain/autism/news/20090511/researchers-see-recovery-from-autism

4. National Vaccine Information Center. (n.d.). About National Vaccine Information Center. Retrieved from www.nvic.org/about.aspx

5. A. Hviid, M. Stellfeld, J. Wohlfahrt, & M. Melbye. (2004). Childhood vaccinations and type I diabetes. *New England Journal of Medicine, 350,* 1398–1404.

6. B. Smith. (2012, February). Dr. Mercola: Visionary or quack? *Chicago Magazine.*

CHAPTER 12

1. K. Reibel. (2008, January 30). Autism and the Amish. Retrieved from http://autism-news-beat.com/archives/29

2. Ibid.

3. Ibid.

4. A. M. Fry et al. (2001). Haemophilus influenzae type b disease among Amish children in Pennsylvania: Reasons for persistent disease. *Pediatrics, 108*(4), E60.

5. G. Harris. (2005, November 8). Five cases of polio in Amish group raise new fears. *New York Times.* Retrieved from www.nytimes.com

6. L. Gostin. (2006). Medical countermeasures for pandemic influenza: Ethics and the law. *Journal of the American Medical Association, 295*(5), 554–556.

7. P. Offit. (2005). Why are pharmaceutical companies gradually abandoning vaccines? *Health Affairs, 24*(3), 622–630.

8. M. Stobbe. (2010, February 7). Millions of swine flu vaccine doses to be burned. *USA Today.* Retrieved from www.usatoday.com

9. A. Berenson. (2005, October 15). Lipitor or generic? Billion dollar battle looms. *New York Times.* Retrieved from www.nytimes.com

10. Offit. (2005).

11. D. E. Sugerman et al. (2010). Measles outbreak in a highly vaccinated population, San Diego 2008: Role of the intentionally undervaccinated. *Pediatrics, 125*(4), 747–755.

12. Domestic Public Health Achievements Team. (2011). Ten great public health achievements: United States 2001–2010. *Morbidity and Mortality Weekly, 60*(19), 619–623.

13. Ibid.

14. National Cancer Institute. (n.d.). NCI health information tip sheet for writers: Cancer health disparities. Retrieved from www.cancer.gov/newscenter/entertainment/tipsheet/cancer-health-disparities

15. Centers for Disease Control and Prevention. (1996). Update: Diphtheria epidemic—new independent states of the former Soviet Union, January 1995–March 1996. *Morbidity and Mortality Weekly, 45*(32), 693–697. Retrieved from www.cdc.gov/mmwr/preview/mmwrhtml/00043378.htm

16. N. Al Dajani & D. Scheifele. (2007). How long can we expect pertussis protection to last after the adolescent booster dose of tetanus-diphtheria-pertussis (TDaP) vaccines? *Paediatrics and Child Health, 12*(10), 873–874.

17. Immunization Action Coalition. (2010). Tetanus disease: Questions and answers. Retrieved from www.vaccineinformation.org/tetanus/qandadis.asp

18. Department of Health and Human Services. (1999, May 18). Testimony on hepatitis B vaccine by Harold S. Margolis, MD. Retrieved from www.hhs.gov/asl/testify/t990518b.html

19. Ibid.

20. Ibid.

21. Ibid.

22. World Health Organization. (2011, July 14). WPRO scarlet fever update. Retrieved from www.wpro.who.int/health_topics/scarlet_fever/

23. National Network for Immunization Information. (2010). Vaccine effectiveness: Do vaccines work? Retrieved from www.immunizationinfo.org/parents/why-immunize

24. Ibid.

25. M. Smith & C. Woods. (2010). On-time vaccine receipt in the first year does not adversely affect neuropsychological outcomes. *Pediatrics, 125*(6), 1134–1141.

26. W. J. Hoyt. (2004). Anti-vaccination fever: The shot hurt around the world. *Skeptical Inquirer, 28*(1). Retrieved from www.csicop.org/si/show/anti-vaccination_fever_the_shot_hurt_around_the_world/

27. Ibid.

28. Ibid.

29. Ibid.

30. Ibid.

31. Ibid.

CHAPTER 13

1. M. Schiffman & P. E. Castle. (2003). Human papillomavirus: Epidemiology and public health. *Archives of Pathology and Laboratory Medicine, 127*(8), 930–934.

2. M. Schiffman, P. E. Castle, J. Jeronimo, A. C. Rodriguez, & S. Wacholder. (2007). Human papillomavirus and cervical cancer. *The Lancet, 370* (9590), 890–907.

3. G. Gross & H. Pfister. (2004). Role of human papillomavirus in penile cancer, penile squamous cell neoplasias and in genital warts. *Medical Microbiology and Immunology, 193*, 35–44.

4. Centers for Disease Control and Prevention. (2011, November 27). Genital HPV infection—fact sheet. Retrieved from www.cdc.gov/std/HPV/STDFact-HPV .htm

5. Ibid.

6. M. A. Goldstein, A. Goodman, M. G. del Carman, & D. C. Wilbur. (2009). Case records of the Massachusetts General Hospital. Case 10-2009. A 23-year-old woman with an abnormal Papanicolaou smear. *New England Journal of Medicine, 360*(13), 1337–1344.

7. Y. Arima et al. (2010). Development of genital warts after incident detection of human papillomavirus infection in young men. *Journal of Infectious Diseases, 202*(8), 1181–1184. doi:10.1086/656368

8. G. Juckett & H. Hartman-Adams. (2010). Human papillomavirus: Clinical manifestations and prevention. *American Family Physician, 82*(10), 1209–1213.

9. J. M. M. Walboomers et al. (1999). Human papillomavirus is a necessary cause of invasive cervical cancer worldwide. *Journal of Pathology, 189*(1), 12–19.

10. Gross & Pfister. (2004).

11. K. K. Ang et al. (2010). Human papillomavirus and survival of patients with oropharyngeal cancer. *New England Journal of Medicine, 363*(1), 24–35. doi:10.1056/ NEJMoa0912217

12. M. C. Stöppler. (2009, April 16). Cervical dysplasia. Retrieved from www .medicinenet.com/cervical_dysplasia/article.htm

13. J. A. Kahn. (2009). HPV vaccination for the prevention of cervical intraepithelial neoplasia. *New England Journal of Medicine, 361*(3), 271–278. doi:10.1056/ NEJMct0806938

14. Reproductive Health Outlook: Cervical Cancer. (n.d.). About cervical cancer. Retrieved from www.rho.org/about-cervical-cancer.htm

15. American Cancer Society. (2011, October 26). What are the key statistics about penile cancer? Retrieved from www.cancer.org/Cancer/PenileCancer/DetailedGuide/ penile-cancer-key-statistics

16. J. Li et al. (2011). Organ-sparing surgery for penile cancer: Complications and outcomes. *Urology, 78*(5), 1121–1124. doi:10.1016/j.urology.2011.08.006

17. B. Schlenker et al. (2011). Intermediate-differentiated invasive (pT1 G2) penile cancer—oncological outcome and follow-up. *Urologic Oncology, 29*(6), 782–787. doi:10.1016/j.urolonc.2009.08.022

18. Centers for Disease Control and Prevention. (2011, November 27).

19. Future II Study Group. (2007). Quadrivalent vaccine against human papillomavirus to prevent high-grade cervical lesions. *New England Journal of Medicine, 356*(19), 1915–1927.

20. B. Hirschler. (2007, February 27). Merck, Sanofi end Gardasil studies due to success. Reuters News Agency. Retrieved from www.reuters.com/article/2007/02/27/idUSL2710961720070227

21. A. L. Goeser. (2007). Quadrivalent HPV recombinant vaccine (Gardasil) for the prevention of cervical cancer. *American Family Physician, 76*(4), 573–574.

22. Centers for Disease Control and Prevention. (2011, December 22). HPV vaccines. Retrieved from www.cdc.gov/hpv/vaccine.html

23. J. Paavonen et al. (2009). Efficacy of human papillomavirus (HPV)-16/18 AS04-adjuvanted vaccine against cervical infection and precancer caused by oncogenic HPV types (PATRICIA): Final analysis of a double-blind, randomised study in young women. *The Lancet, 374*(9686), 301–314. doi:10.1016/S0140-6736(09)61248-4

24. M. Gaul. (2006, February 6). Family Research Council statement regarding HPV vaccines. Retrieved from www.nccc-online.org/health_news/topics/controversial/family_research.html

25. L. A. Johnson. (2007, February 21). Merck suspends lobbying for vaccine. *Washington Post.* Retrieved from www.washingtonpost.com

26. Associated Press. (2007, February 3). Texas governor orders STD vaccine for all girls. Retrieved from www.msnbc.msn.com/id/16948093/ns/health-childrens_health/t/texas-governor-orders-std-vaccine-all-girls/#.Tw8DzNWaUlc

27. Texas House of Representatives. HB 1098. Retrieved from www.legis.state.tx.us/tlodocs/80R/billtext/html/HB01098F.htm

28. J. Terbush. (2011, September 13). Does the HPV vaccine really cause retardation? *Business Insider.* Retrieved from www.businessinsider.com

29. M. Herper. (2011, September 15). Bioethicist offers $10,000 reward for proof of Bachmann vaccine claims. *Forbes.* Retrieved from www.forbes.com

30. J. Hafner. (2011, November 14). To one Iowa mother, Bachmann decries "the ravages" of HPV vaccine. *Des Moines Register.* Retrieved from www.caucuses.desmoinesregister.com

31. L. W. Kang et al. (2008). Hypersensitivity reactions to human papillomavirus vaccine in Australian schoolgirls: Retrospective cohort study. *British Medical Journal, 337*(7683), 1392.

32. J. M. Brotherton et al. (2008). Anaphylaxis following quadrivalent human papillomavirus vaccination. *Canadian Medical Association Journal, 279*(6), 525–533.

33. National Vaccine Information Center. (2009, February). An analysis by the National Vaccine Information Center of Gardasil and Menactra adverse event reports to the Vaccine Adverse Events Reporting System (VAERS). Retrieved from www.nvic.org/Downloads/NVICGardasilvsMenactraVAERSReportFeb-2009u.aspx

34. Merck & Co., Inc. (2009, January 9). Merck & Co., Inc. receives complete response letter from the Food and Drug Administration for use of Gardasil in women ages 27 through 45. Retrieved from www.businesswire.com

35. Ibid.

36. R. Chitale. (2009, August 19). CDC report stirs controversy for Merck's Gardasil vaccine. *ABC News.* Retrieved from www.abcnews.go.com

37. J. L. Brotherton, M. Fridman, C. L. May, G. Chappell, A. Saville, & D. M. Gertig. (2011). Early effect of the HPV vaccination programme on cervical abnormalities in Victoria, Australia: An ecological study. *The Lancet, 377*(9783), 2085–2092.

38. Ibid.

39. National Cervical Cancer Coalition. (n.d.). What is the National Cervical Cancer Coalition? Retrieved from www.nccc-online.org/

CHAPTER 14

1. BBC News Health. (2011, December 2). WHO issues Europe measles warning. Retrieved from www.bbc.co.uk

Bibliography

Advisory Committee on Immunization Practices. (1998). Measles, mumps and rubella—vaccine use and strategies for elimination of measles, rubella and congenital rubella syndrome and control of mumps: Recommendation of the advisory committee on immunization practices. *Morbidity and Mortality Weekly, 47*(RR-8), 1–57.

Al Dajani, N., & Scheifele, D. (2007). How long can we expect pertussis protection to last after the adolescent booster dose of tetanus-diphtheria-pertussis (TDaP) vaccines? *Paediatrics and Child Health, 12*(10), 873–874.

Allen, A. (2007). *Vaccine: The controversial story of medicine's greatest lifesaver.* New York: Norton.

Alm, J. S., Lilja, G., Pershagen, G., & Scheynius, A. (1997). Early BCG vaccination and development of atopy. *The Lancet, 350*(9075), 400–403.

American Academy of Child and Adolescent Psychiatry. (2011, March). Facts for families: Obesity in children and teens. Retrieved from www.aacap.org/galleries/FactsForFamilies/79_obesity_in_children_and_teens.pdf

American Academy of Pediatrics. (2011, January 20). What parents should know about measles-mumps-rubella (MMR) vaccine and autism. Retrieved from www2.aap.org/immunization/families/autismfacts.html

American Academy of Pediatrics. (n.d.). Why immunize? Retrieved from www2.aap.org/immunization/families/whyimmunize.html

American Cancer Society. (2011, October 26). What are the key statistics about penile cancer? Retrieved from www.cancer.org/Cancer/PenileCancer/DetailedGuide/penile-cancer-key-statistics

American Psychiatric Association. (2000). Autism. *Diagnostic and statistical manual of mental disorders: DSM-IV-TR* (4th ed.). Washington, DC: American Psychiatric Association.

Anderson, H. R., Poloniecki, J. D., Strachan, D. P., Beasley, R., Bjorksten, B., & Asher, M. I. (2001). Immunization and symptoms of atopic disease in children: Results from the international study of asthma and allergies in childhood. *American Journal of Public Health, 91*(7), 1126–1129.

Anderson, R. M., & May, R. M. (1985). Vaccination and herd immunity to infectious diseases. *Nature, 318*, 323–329.

Andrews, N., Miller, E., Grant, A., Stowe, J., Osborn, V., & Taylor, B. (2004). Thimerosal exposure in infants and developmental disorders: A retrospective cohort study in the United Kingdom does not support a causal association. *Pediatrics, 114*, 584–591. doi:10.1542/peds.2003-1177-L

Ang, K. K., et al. (2010). Human papillomavirus and survival of patients with oropharyngeal cancer. *New England Journal of Medicine, 363*(1), 24–35. doi:10.1056/NEJMoa0912217

Anonymous. (2010). Retraction: Ileal-lymphoid-nodular hyperplasia, non-specific colitis, and pervasive developmental disorder in children. *The Lancet, 375*(9713), 445.

Anonymous. (2011, August 25). Hemoglobin: Magical colors of the power red. Stanford School of Medicine Blood Center. Retrieved from http://bloodcenter.stanford.edu/blog/archives/2011/08/magical-powers.html

Arima, Y., et al. (2010). Development of genital warts after incident detection of human papillomavirus infection in young men. *Journal of Infectious Diseases, 202*(8), 1181–1184. doi:10.1086/656368

Arking, D., et al. (2008). Association between microdeletion and microduplication at 16p11.2 and autism. *New England Journal of Medicine, 358*(7), 667–675.

Arora, P., et al. (2011). Genetic polymorphisms of innate immunity-related inflammatory pathways and their association with factors related to type 2 diabetes. *BMC Medical Genetics, 12*(1), 95–103. doi:10.1186/1471-2350-12-95

Asif Doja, A., & Roberts, W. (2006). Immunizations and autism: A review of the literature. *Canadian Journal of Neurological Sciences, 33*(4), 341–346.

Associated Press. (2007, February 3). Texas governor orders STD vaccine for all girls. Retrieved from www.msnbc.msn.com/id/16948093/ns/health-childrens_health/t/texas-governor-orders-std-vaccine-all-girls/#.Tw8DzNWaUlc

Asthma and Allergy Foundation of America. (n.d.). Allergy facts and figures. Retrieved from www.aafa.org/display.cfm?id=9&sub=30#_ftnref1

Atkinson, R. L. (2007). Viruses as an etiology of obesity. *Mayo Clinic Proceedings, 82*(10), 1192–1198.

Atladóttir, H., et al. (2010). Maternal infection requiring hospitalization during pregnancy and autism spectrum disorders. *Journal of Autism and Developmental Disorders, 40*(12), 1423–1430.

Banaschewski, T., Becker, K., Scherag, S., Franke, B., & Coghill, D. (2010). Molecular genetics of attention-deficit/hyperactivity disorder: An overview. *European Child and Adolescent Psychiatry, 19*(3), 237–257. doi:10.1007/s00787-010-0090-z

Banerjee, T., Middleton, F., & Faraone, S. V. (2007). Environmental risk factors for attention-deficit hyperactivity disorder. *Acta Paediatrica, 96*(9), 1269–1274. doi:10.1111/j.1651-2227.2007.00430.x

Barkely, R. A. (2000). Genetics of childhood disorders: XVII. ADHD, part I: The executive functions and ADHD. *Journal of the American Academy of Child and Adolescent Psychiatry, 39*(8), 1064–1068.

Barquet, N., & Domingo, P. (1997). Smallpox: The triumph over the most terrible of the ministers of death. *Annals of Internal Medicine, 127*(8:1), 635–642.

Barrett, S. (2003, October 9). Dr. Mark Geier severely criticized. Retrieved from www.casewatch.org/civil/geier.shtml

Barrett, S., & Baratz, R. S. (2005, April 20). Disciplinary actions against Herman Hugh Fudenberg, M.D. Retrieved from www.casewatch.org/board/med/fudenberg/1995order.shtml

Baxter, A. J., & Krenzelok, E. P. (2008). Pediatric fatality secondary to EDTA chelation. *Clinical Toxicology, 46,* 1083–1084. doi:10.1080/15563650701261488

BBC News Health. (2011, December 2). WHO issues Europe measles warning. Retrieved from www.bbc.co.uk

Beauchamp, R. A., et al. (2006). Deaths associated with hypocalcemia from chelation therapy: Texas, Pennsylvania, and Oregon, 2003–2005. *Journal of the American Medical Association, 295*(18), 2131–2133.

Berenson, A. (2005, October 15). Lipitor or generic? Billion dollar battle looms. *New York Times.* Retrieved from www.nytimes.com

Bernard, S., Enayati, A., Redwood, L., Roger, H., & Binstock, T. (2001). Autism: A novel form of mercury poisoning. *Medical Hypotheses, 56*(4), 462–471. doi:10.1054/mehy.2000.1281

Bijanzadeh, M., Mahesh, P. A., & Ramachand, N. B. (2011). An understanding of the genetic basis of asthma. *Indian Journal of Medical Research, 134*(2), 149–161.

Black, C., Kaye, J. A., & Jick, H. (2002). Relation of childhood gastrointestinal disorders to autism: Nested case-control study using data from the UK General Practice Research Database. *British Medical Journal, 325*(7361), 419–421.

Booth, M. (2011, November 29). Colorado parents rank second in nation for vaccine refusals. *Denver Post.* Retrieved from www.denverpost.com

Bornovalova, M., Hicks, B., Iacono, W., & McGue, M. (2010). Familial transmission and heritability of childhood disruptive disorders. *American Journal of Psychiatry, 167*(9), 1066–1074.

Bradfield, J. P., et al. (2011). A genome-wide meta-analysis of six type 1 diabetes cohorts identifies multiple associated loci. *PLoS Genetics, 7*(9), 1–8. doi:10.1371/journal.pgen.1002293

Brotherton, J. L., Fridman, M., May, C. L., Chappell, G., Saville, A., & Gertig, D. M. (2011). Early effect of the HPV vaccination programme on cervical abnormalities in Victoria, Australia: An ecological study. *The Lancet, 377*(9783), 2085–2092.

Brotherton, J. M., Gold, M. S., Kemp, A. S., McIntyre, P. B., Burgess, M. A., & Campbell-Lloyd, S. (2008). Anaphylaxis following quadrivalent human papillomavirus vaccination. *Canadian Medical Association Journal, 279*(6), 525–533.

Bumble Bee Foods, LLC. (n.d.). Current topics. Retrieved from www.bumblebee.com/faqs

Burney, P. J., Newson, R. B., Burrows, M. S., & Wheeler, D. M. (2008). The effects of allergens in outdoor air on both atopic and nonatopic subjects with airway disease. *Allergy, 63*(5), 542–546. doi:10.1111/j.1398-9995.2007.01596.x

Calonge, N. (2008, March 30). Fear over vaccines and autism: No science behind recent scare. *Denver Post.* Retrieved from www.denverpost.com

Carr, K. (2011, October 21). Smallpox. Retrieved from www.historyforkids.org/learn/science/medicine/smallpox.htm

Carter, T. (2004, November 18). *MMR: What they didn't tell you.* London: Channel 4.

Case, C., & Chung, K. (1997). Montagu and Jenner: The campaign against smallpox. *SIM News, 47*(2), 58–60.

Center for Food Safety. (2009, May 1). Risk in brief: Formaldehyde in food. The Government of the Hong Kong Special Administrative Region. Retrieved from www.cfs .gov.hk/english/programme/programme_rafs/programme_rafs_fa_02_09.html

Centers for Disease Control and Prevention. (1990). Current trends tetanus—United States, 1987 and 1988. *Morbidity and Mortality Weekly, 39*(3), 37–41.

Centers for Disease Control and Prevention. (1996). Update: Diphtheria epidemic— new independent states of the former Soviet Union, January 1995–March 1996. *Morbidity and Mortality Weekly, 45*(32), 693–697.

Centers for Disease Control and Prevention. (1999). Withdrawal of rotavirus vaccine recommendation. *Morbidity and Mortality Weekly, 48*(43), 1007.

Centers for Disease Control and Prevention. (2003). History and epidemiology of global smallpox eradication. [PowerPoint slides]. Retrieved from www.bt.cdc.gov/ agent/smallpox/training/overview/pdf/eradicationhistory.pdf

Centers for Disease Control and Prevention. (2004, December 30). Smallpox disease overview. Retrieved from www.bt.cdc.gov/agent/smallpox/overview/disease-facts.asp

Centers for Disease Control and Prevention. (2009, August 31). Complications of measles. Retrieved from www.cdc.gov/measles/about/complications.html

Centers for Disease Control and Prevention. (2010, February 12). Update: Mumps outbreak New York and New Jersey, June 2009–January 2010. *Morbidity and Mortality Weekly Report, 59*(5), 125–129.

Centers for Disease Control and Prevention. (2011). Vaccine excipient and media summary. In Atkinson, W., Wolfe, S., & Hamborsky, J. (Eds.). *Epidemiology and prevention of vaccine-preventable diseases* (12th ed.). Washington, DC: Public Health Foundation. Retrieved from www.cdc.gov/vaccines/pubs/pinkbook/down loads/appendices/B/excipient-table-1.pdf

Centers for Disease Control and Prevention. (2011, March 11). Meningitis: Questions and answers. Retrieved from www.cdc.gov/meningitis/about/faq.html

Centers for Disease Control and Prevention. (2011, April 21). Possible side-effects from vaccines. Retrieved from www.cdc.gov/vaccines/vac-gen/side-effects.htm

Centers for Disease Control and Prevention. (2011, May 27). Measles—United States, January–May 20, 2011. *Morbidity and Mortality Weekly, 60*(20), 666–668.

Centers for Disease Control and Prevention. (2011, June 24). What would happen if we stopped vaccinations? Retrieved from www.cdc.gov/vaccines/vac-gen/ whatifstop.htm

Centers for Disease Control and Prevention. (2011, June 29). Measles: Make sure your child is fully immunized. Retrieved from www.cdc.gov/features/measles/

Centers for Disease Control and Prevention. (2011, August 4). Hepatitis A FAQs for health officials. Retrieved from www.cdc.gov/hepatitis/HAV/HAVfaq.htm

Centers for Disease Control and Prevention. (2011, August 22). Pertussis (whooping cough) outbreaks. Retrieved from www.cdc.gov/pertussis/outbreaks.html

Centers for Disease Control and Prevention. (2011, October 27). Human papillomavirus (HPV). Retrieved from www.cdc.gov/hpv/

Centers for Disease Control and Prevention. (2011, November 27). Genital HPV infection—fact sheet. Retrieved from www.cdc.gov/std/hpv/stdfact-hpv.htm

Centers for Disease Control and Prevention. (2011, December 1). Pneumonia can be prevented: Vaccines can help. Retrieved from www.cdc.gov/Features/Pneumonia/

Centers for Disease Control and Prevention. (2011, December 22). HPV vaccines. Retrieved from www.cdc.gov/hpv/vaccine.html

Chabris, C., & Simons, D. (2011). *The invisible gorilla: How our intuitions deceive us.* New York: Broadway.

Chandan, J. V., Bunge, S. A., Dudukovic, N. M., Zalecki, C. A., Elliot, G. R., & Gabrielli, J. D. E. (2005). Altered neural substrates of cognitive control in childhood ADHD: Evidence from functional magnetic resonance imaging. *American Journal of Psychiatry, 162*(9), 1605–1613.

Chen, S., Maeda, T., Yoichi, S., Yamagata, Z., Tomiwa, K., & Japan Children's Study Group. (2010). Early television exposure and children's behavioral and social outcomes at age 30 months. *Journal of Epidemiology, 20*(Suppl. 2), S482–S489. doi:10.2188/jea.JE20090179

Cherry, D. (1999). Pertussis in the pre-antibiotic and pre-vaccine era with an emphasis on adult pertussis. *Clinical Infectious Diseases, 28,* S107–S111.

Cheslack-Postava, K., Liu, K., & Bearman, P. S. (2011). Closely spaced pregnancies are associated with increased odds of autism in California sibling births. *Pediatrics, 127*(2), 246–253.

Chitale, R. (2009, August 19). CDC report stirs controversy for Merck's Gardasil vaccine. *ABC News.* Retrieved from www.abcnews.go.com

Christakis, D. A., Zimmerman, F. J., DiGiuseppe, D. L., & McCarty, C. A. (2004). Early television exposure and subsequent attentional problems in children. *Pediatrics, 113,* 708–713.

Classen, D. C., & Classen, J. B. (1997). The timing of pediatric immunization and the risk of insulin-dependent diabetes mellitus. *Infectious Diseases in Clinical Practice, 6*(7), 449–454.

Classen, J. B., & Classen, D. C. (1999). Vertically transmitted enteroviruses and the benefits of neonatal immunization. *Diabetes Care, 22*(10), 1760–1761.

Cohn, M. (2011, May 19). Son of autism doctor charged with practicing without a license. *Baltimore Sun.* Retrieved from www.baltimoresun.com

Cook Jr., E. H. (1999). Genetics of attention-deficit hyperactivity disorder. *Mental Retardation and Developmental Disabilities Research Reviews, 5*(3), 191–198.

Courchesne, E., et al. (2011). Neuron number and size in prefrontal cortex of children with autism. *Journal of the American Medical Association, 306*(18), 2001–2010.

Courvoisie, H., Hooper, S. R., Fine, C., Kwock, L., & Castillo, M. (2004). Neurometabolic functioning and neuropsychological correlates in children with ADHD-H: Preliminary findings. *Journal of Neuropsychiatry and Clinical Neurosciences, 16,* 63–69.

Cox, D. J., Kovatchev, B. P., Morris, J. B., Phillips, C., Hill, R. J., & Merkel, L. (1998). Electroencephalographic and psychometric differences between boys with and without attention-deficit/hyperactivity disorder (ADHD): A pilot study. *Applied Psychophysiology and Biofeedback, 23*(3), 179–188.

Curns, A. T., Steiner, C. A., Barrett, M., Hunter, K., Wilson, E., & Parashar, U. D. (2010). Reduction in acute gastroenteritis hospitalizations among US children after introduction of rotavirus vaccine: Analysis of hospital discharge data from 18 states. *Journal of Infectious Diseases, 201,* 1617–1624.

Dales, L., Hammer, S. J., & Smith, N. J. (2001). Time trends in autism and in MMR immunization coverage in California. *Journal of the American Medical Association, 285*(9), 1183–1185.

Daniels, J., et al. (2008). Parental psychiatric disorders associated with autism spectrum disorders in the offspring. *Pediatrics, 121*(5), E1357.

Davis, M., Patel, M., & Gebremariam, A. (2004). Decline in varicella-related hospitalizations and expenditures for children and adults after introduction of varicella vaccine in the United States. *Pediatrics, 114*(3), 786–792.

Deer, B. (2006, December 31). MMR scare doctor got legal aid fortune. *Sunday Times* (London). Record number 908788052.

Deer, B. (2011a). How the case against the MMR vaccine was fixed. *British Medical Journal, 342,* 77–82. doi:10.1136/bmj.c5347

Deer, B. (2011b). How the vaccine crisis was meant to make money. *British Medical Journal, 342*(7789). 136–142. doi:10.1136/bmj.c5258

Deer, B. (2011, July 22). Revealed: Wakefield's secret first MMR patent claims "safer measles vaccine." Retrieved from http:briandeer.com/wakefield/vaccine-patent.htm

Deer, B. (2011, August 4). Royal Free facilitates attack on MMR in medical school single shots videotape. Retrieved from http:briandeer.com/wakefield/royal-video.htm

Deer, B. (2011, August 5). Royal Free autism pill partner, Herman Hugh Fudenberg, wasn't fit to prescribe. Retrieved from http:briandeer.com/wakefield/hugh-fudenberg.htm

Demirci, C. S., & Abuhammour, W. (2011, November 23). Pediatric diphtheria. Medscape: Drugs, diseases and procedures. Retrieved from emedicine.medscape.com/article/963334-overview

Department of Health and Human Services. (1999, May 18). Testimony on hepatitis B vaccine by Harold S. Margolis, MD. Retrieved from www.hhs.gov/asl/testify/t990518b.html

DeStefano, F., Bhasin, T. K., Thompson, W. W., Yeargin-Allsopp, M., & Boyle, C. (2004). Age at first measles-mumps-rubella vaccination in children with autism and school-matched control subjects: A population-based study in metropolitan Atlanta. *Pediatrics, 113*(2), 259–266.

DeStefano, F., et al. (2002). Childhood vaccinations and risk of asthma. *Pediatric Infectious Disease Journal, 21,* 498–504. doi:10.1097/00006454-200206000-00004

Dire, D. (2011, September 20). Tetanus in emergency medicine. Retrieved from http:emedicine.medscape.com/article/786414-overview#a0199

Doheny, K. (2009, May 11). Researchers see recovery from autism: Study shows some children may "move off" the autistic spectrum. WebMD Health News. Retrieved from www.webmd.com/brain/autism/news/20090511/researchers-see-recovery-from-autism

Domestic Public Health Achievements Team. (2011). Ten great public health achievements: United States 2001–2010. *Morbidity and Mortality Weekly, 60*(19), 619–623.

Dominus, S. (2011, April 24). The crash and burn of an autism guru. *New York Times.* Retrieved from www.nytimes.com

Downshen, S. (2009, November). Smallpox. Retrieved from http://kidshealth.org/teen/infections/skin_rashes/smallpox.html#

Eick, A. A., et al. (2011). Maternal influenza vaccination and effect on influenza virus infection in young infants. *Archives of Pediatric and Adolescent Medicine, 165*(2), 104–111. doi:10.1001/archpediatrics.2010.192

Eickhorn, T. C. (2008). Penicillin: An accidental discovery changed the course of medicine. *Endocrine Today.* Retrieved from www.endocrinetoday.com/view.aspx?rid=30176

Ekbom, A., Daszak, P., Kraaz, W., & Wakefield, A. J. (1996). Crohn's disease after in-utero measles virus exposure. *The Lancet, 348*(9026), 515–517.

Elliman, D. (1999). Vaccination and type 1 diabetes mellitus: Currently no evidence of a link, but more studies are needed as vaccines change. *British Medical Journal, 318*(7192), 1159–1160.

Ellman, L. M., et al. (2010). Structural brain alterations in schizophrenia following fetal exposure to the inflammatory cytokine interleukin-8. *Schizophrenia Research, 121*(1–3), 46–54.

Environmental Working Group. (n.d.). 2011 shopper's guide to pesticides in produce. Retrieved from www.ewg.org/foodnews/

Finsen, N. R. (1895). The red light treatment of small-pox. *British Medical Journal, 2*(1823), 1412–1414.

Finucane, M., et al. (2011). National, regional, and global trends in body-mass index since 1980: Systematic analysis of health examination surveys and epidemiological studies with 960 country-years and 9.1 million participants. *The Lancet, 377*(9765), 557–567.

Flanders, J. (2005). *Inside the Victorian home: A portrait of domestic life in Victorian England.* New York: Norton.

Fletcher, B., Gulanick, M., & Lamendola, C. (2002). Risk factors for type 2 diabetes mellitus. *Journal of Cardiovascular Nursing, 16*(2), 17–23.

Fombonne, E., & Chakrabarti, S. (2001). No evidence for a new variant of measles-mumps-rubella-induced autism. *Pediatrics, 108*(4), E58. doi:10.1542/peds.108.4.e58

Fombonne, E., Zakarian, R., Bennett, A., Meng, L., & McLean-Heywood, D. (2006). Pervasive developmental disorders in Montreal, Quebec, Canada: Prevalence and links with immunizations. *Pediatrics 118*(1), E139–E150; doi:10.1542/peds.2005-2993

Food Standards Australia New Zealand. (2003, June). Sodium glutamate: A safety assessment. Retrieved from www.foodstandards.gov.au/_srcfiles/MSG%20Technical%20Report.pdf

Fry, A. M., et al. (2001). Haemophilus influenzae type b disease among Amish children in Pennsylvania: Reasons for persistent disease. *Pediatrics, 108*(4), E60.

Future II Study Group. (2007). Quadrivalent vaccine against human papillomavirus to prevent high-grade cervical lesions. *New England Journal of Medicine, 356*(19), 1915–1927.

Gaul, M. (2006, February 6). Family Research Council statement regarding HPV vaccines. Retrieved from www.nccc-online.org/health_news/topics/controversial/family_research.html

Geier, D. A., & Geier, M. R. (2002). Serious neurological conditions following pertussis immunization: An analysis of endotoxin levels, the Vaccine Adverse Events Reporting System (VAERS) database and literature review. *Pediatric Rehabilitation, 5*(3), 177–182. doi:10.1080/1363849021000054031

Geier, D. A., & Geier, M. R. (2003). An assessment of the impact of thimerosal on childhood neurodevelopmental disorders. *Pediatric Rehabilitation, 6*(2), 97. doi:10.1080/1363849031000139315

Geier, D. A., & Geier, M. R. (2004a). An evaluation of serious neurological disorders following immunization: A comparison of whole-cell pertussis and acellular pertussis vaccines. *Brain and Development, 26*(5), 296–300. doi:10.1016/S0387-7604(03)00169-4

Geier, D. A., & Geier, M. R. (2004b). Neurodevelopmental disorders following thimerosal-containing childhood immunizations: A follow-up analysis. *International Journal of Toxicology, 23*(6), 369–376. doi:10.1080/10915810490902038

Geier, D. A., & Geier, M. R. (2005). A case-control study of serious autoimmune adverse events following hepatitis B immunization. *Autoimmunity, 38*(4), 295–301. doi:10.1080/08916930500144484

Geier, D. A., & Geier, M. R. (2006). An evaluation of the effects of thimerosal on neurodevelopmental disorders reported following DTP and Hib vaccines in comparison to DTPH vaccine in the United States. *Journal of Toxicology and Environmental Health: Part A, 69*(15), 1481–1495. doi:10.1080/15287390500364556

Geier, M. R., & Geier, D. A. (2005). The potential importance of steroids in the treatment of autistic spectrum disorders and other disorders involving mercury toxicity. *Medical Hypotheses, 64*(5), 946–954. doi:10.1016/j.mehy.2004.11.018

Geier, M. R., Geier, D. A., & Zahalsky, A. C. (2003). Influenza vaccination and Guillain-Barre syndrome. *Clinical Immunology, 107*(2), 116. doi:10.1016/S1521-6616(03)00046-9

General Medical Council. (2010, May 24). Determination on serious professional misconduct (SPM) and sanction. Retrieved from www.gmc-uk.org/Wakefield_SPM_and_SANCTION.pdf_32595267.pdf

Gernsbacher, M. S., Dawson, M., & Goldsmith, H. H. (2005). Three reasons not to believe in an autism epidemic. *Current Directions in Psychological Science, 14*, 55–58. doi:10.1111/j.0963-7214.2005.00334.x

Goeser, A. L. (2007). Quadrivalent HPV recombinant vaccine (Gardasil) for the prevention of cervical cancer. *American Family Physician, 76*(4), 573–574.

Goldstein, M. A., Goodman, A., del Carman, M. G., & Wilbur, D. C. (2009). Case records of the Massachusetts General Hospital. Case 10-2009. A 23-year-old woman with an abnormal Papanicolaou smear. *New England Journal of Medicine, 360*(13), 1337–1344.

Goodman, M. J., & Nordin, J. (2006). Vaccine Adverse Event Reporting System reporting source: A possible source of bias in longitudinal studies. *Pediatrics, 117*(2), 387–390. doi:10.1542/peds.2004-2687

Gostin, L. (2006). Medical countermeasures for pandemic influenza: Ethics and the law. *Journal of the American Medical Association, 295*(5), 554–556.

Greger, M. (2006). *Bird flu: A virus of our own hatching.* Lantern Books. Retrieved from http:birdflubook.com/a.php?id=40

Gross, G., & Pfister, H. (2004). Role of human papillomavirus in penile cancer, penile squamous cell neoplasias and in genital warts. *Medical Microbiology and Immunology, 193,* 35–44.

Hafner, J. (2011, November 14). To one Iowa mother, Bachmann decries "the ravages" of HPV vaccine. *Des Moines Register.* Retrieved from www.caucuses .desmoinesregister.com

Halsall, P. (Ed.). (1998, July). Modern history sourcebook: Lady Mary Wortley Montagu (1689–1762): Smallpox vaccination in Turkey. Fordham University Internet History Sourcebooks Project. Retrieved from www.fordham.edu/halsall/ mod/montagu-smallpox.asp

Harris, G. (2005, November 8). Five cases of polio in Amish group raise new fears. *New York Times.* Retrieved from www.nytimes.com

Harvard Center for Risk Analysis. (2009). Causes of death. Harvard School of Public Health. Retrieved from www.hcra.harvard.edu/quiz.html

Heilprin, J. (2011, April 21). Measles outbreak in Europe, especially France. *Huffington Post.* Retrieved from www.huffingtonpost.com

Henderson, D. A., & Preston, R. (2009). *Smallpox—the death of a disease: The inside story of eradicating a worldwide killer.* Amherst, NY: Prometheus Books.

Hepatitis B Foundation. (2009, October 21). About hepatitis B: Statistics. Retrieved from www.hepb.org/hepb/statistics.htm

Heron, J., & Golden, J. (2004). Thimerosal exposure in infants and developmental disorders: A prospective cohort study in the United Kingdom does not support a causal association. *Pediatrics, 114*(3), 577.

Herper, M. (2011, September 15). Bioethicist offers $10,000 reward for proof of Bachmann vaccine claims. *Forbes.* Retrieved from www.forbes.com

Hertz-Picciotto, I., Green, P., Delwiche, L., Hansen, R., Walker, C., & Pessah, I. (2010). Blood mercury concentrations in CHARGE Study children with and without autism. *Environmental Health Perspectives, 118*(1), 161–166. doi:10.1289/ehp.0900736

Hirschler, B. (2007, February 27). Merck, Sanofi end Gardasil studies due to success. Reuters News Agency. Retrieved from www.reuters.com/article/2007/02/27/ idUSL2710961720070227

Hoekstra, R. A., Bartels, M., Verweij, C. J. H., & Boomsma, D. I. (2007). Heritability of autistic traits in the general population. *Archives of Pediatric and Adolescent Medicine, 161,* 372–377.

Hopkins, D. R. (1983). *Princes and peasants: Smallpox in history.* Chicago: University of Chicago Press.

Hopkins, D. R. (2002). *The greatest killer: Smallpox in history.* Chicago: University of Chicago Press.

Hornig, M., et al. (2008). Lack of association between measles virus vaccine and autism with enteropathy: A case-control study. *PLoS One, 3*(9), E3140. doi:10.1371/journal.pone.0003140

Hostess Brands, Inc. (n.d.). Wonder Smartwhite bread. Retrieved from www.wonder bread.com/white-bread.html

Hoyt, W. J. (2004). Anti-vaccination fever: The shot hurt around the world. *Skeptical Inquirer, 28*(1). Retrieved from www.csicop.org/si/show/anti-vaccination_fever_the_shot_hurt_around_the_world/

Hunt, M. (2011, May 24). Rubella (German measles) virus. Microbiology and Immunology On-line. University of South Carolina School of Medicine. Retrieved from http:pathmicro.med.sc.edu/mhunt/rubella.htm

Hviid, A., Stellfeld, M., Wohlfahrt, J., & Melbye, M. (2004). Childhood vaccinations and type I diabetes. *New England Journal of Medicine, 350,* 1398–1404.

Immunization Action Coalition. (2010). Tetanus disease: Questions and answers. Retrieved from www.vaccineinformation.org/tetanus/qandadis.asp

Immunization Action Coalition. (2011, March). Hib disease: Questions and answers. Retrieved from www.vaccineinformation.org/hib/qandadis.asp

Institute for Vaccine Safety. (2011, June 13). Components of vaccines. Johns Hopkins Bloomberg School of Public Health. Retrieved from www.vaccinesafety.edu/components.htm

Institute for Vaccine Safety. (2011, October 3). Components of DTaP vaccine. Johns Hopkins Bloomberg School of Public Health. Retrieved from www.vaccinesafety.edu/components-DTaP.htm

Institute for Vaccine Safety. (2011, October 3). Components of MMR vaccines. Johns Hopkins Bloomberg School of Public Health. Retrieved from www.vaccine safety.edu/components-MMR.htm

Institute for Vaccine Safety. (2011, October 3). Components of seasonal influenza vaccines. Johns Hopkins Bloomberg School of Public Health. Retrieved from www.vaccinesafety.edu/components-Influenza.htm

Institute for Vaccine Safety. (2011, October 10). Components of DTaP, hep B and IPV vaccine. Johns Hopkins Bloomberg School of Public Health. Retrieved from www.vaccinesafety.edu/components-DTaP-HepB-IPV.htm

Institute of Medicine. (2001). Frequently asked questions: Measles-mumps-rubella vaccine and autism. Retrieved from www.iom.edu/~/media/Files/Report%20 Files/2003/Immunization-Safety-Review-Measles-Mumps-Rubella-Vaccine-and-Autism/MMRFAQ2pager.pdf

Institute of Medicine. (2001). Frequently asked questions: Thimerosal in vaccines. Retrieved from iom.edu/~/media/Files/Report%20Files/2003/Immunization-Safety-Review-Thimerosal---Containing-Vaccines-and-Neurodevelopmental-Disorders/ThimerosalFAQ.pdf

Institute of Medicine. (2004). *Immunization safety review: Vaccines and autism.* Washington, DC: National Academies Press.

Jefferson, T., & Demicheli, V. (1998). No evidence that vaccines cause insulin-dependent diabetes mellitus. *Journal of Epidemiology and Community Health, 52*(10), 674–675.

Jefferson, T., Rudin, M., & DiPietrantonj, C. (2004). Adverse events after immunisation with aluminium-containing DTP vaccines: Systematic review of the evidence. *The Lancet Infectious Diseases, 4*(2), 84–90.

Johnson, A. (2009, February 13). U.S. court rejects vaccine connection to autism. *Wall Street Journal.* Retrieved from www.online.wsj.com

Johnson, C. E., Whitwell, J., Kumar, M. L., Nalin, D. R., Chui, L. W., & Marusyk, R. G. (1994). Measles vaccine immunogenicity in 6-versus 15-month-old infants born to mothers in the measles vaccine era. *Pediatrics, 93*(6), 939–942.

Johnson, L. A. (2007, February 21). Merck suspends lobbying for vaccine. *Washington Post.* Retrieved from www.washingtonpost.com

Juckett, G., & Hartman-Adams, H. (2010). Human papillomavirus: Clinical manifestations and prevention. *American Family Physician, 82*(10), 1209–1213.

Kahn, J. A. (2009). HPV vaccination for the prevention of cervical intraepithelial neoplasia. *New England Journal of Medicine, 361*(3), 271–278. doi:10.1056/NEJMct0806938

Kang, L., et al. (2008). Hypersensitivity reactions to human papillomavirus vaccine in Australian schoolgirls: Retrospective cohort study. *British Medical Journal, 337*(7683), 1392.

Kaplowitz, P. B., Speiser, P. W., Windle, M. L., Levitsky, L. L., Poth, M. P. M., & Kemp, S. (2010, March 29). Precocious puberty. Retrieved from http:emedicine.medscape.com/article/924002-overview

Kaye, J. A., del Mar Melero-Montes, M., & Jick, H. (2001). Mumps, measles, and rubella vaccine and the incidence of autism recorded by general practitioners: A time trend analysis. *British Medical Journal, 322,* 460. doi:10.1136/bmj.322.7284.460

Kemner, C., Jonkman, L. M., Kenemans, J. L., Bocker, K. B. E., Verbaten, M. N., & van Engeland, H. (2004). Sources of auditory selective attention and the effects of methylphenidate in children with attention-deficit/hyperactivity disorder. *Biological Psychiatry, 55,* 776–778.

Kim, B., Lee, J., Shin, M., Cho, S., & Lee, D. (2002). Regional cerebral perfusion abnormalities in attention deficit/hyperactivity disorder: Statistical parametric mapping analysis. *European Archives of Psychiatry and Clinical Neuroscience, 252*(5), 219.

Klein, J. (2009, September). Rotavirus. Retrieved from http:kidshealth.org/parent/infections/stomach/rotavirus.html#

Klein, J. (2010, September). Polio. Kids Health. Retrieved from http:kidshealth.org/parent/infections/bacterial_viral/polio.html#

Klein, K. D., & Diehl, E. G. (2004). Relationship between MMR vaccine and autism. *Annals of Pharmacotherapy, 38*(7–8), 1297–1300.

Knox, R. (2005, October 5). 1918 killer flu reconstructed. National Public Radio. Retrieved from www.npr.org/templates/story/story.php?storyId=4946718

Kolevzon, A., Gross, R., & Reichenberg, A. (2007). Prenatal and perinatal risk factors for autism. *Archives of Pediatric and Adolescent Medicine, 161,* 326–333.

Kuehn, B. M. (2010). Increased risk of ADHD associated with early exposure to pesticides, PCBs. *Journal of the American Medical Association, 304*(1), 27–28.

Laidler, J. R. (2005, July 27). Chelation and autism. *Neurodiversity weblog.* Retrieved from http:neurodiversity.com/weblog/article/14/chelation-autism

Leblanc, S. (2007, October 18). Parents use religion to avoid vaccines. *USA Today*. Retrieved from www.usatoday.com

Li, J., et al. (2011). Organ-sparing surgery for penile cancer: Complications and outcomes. *Urology, 78*(5), 1121–1124. doi:10.1016/j.urology.2011.08.006

Limperopoulos, C. J. (2007). Does cerebral injury in premature infants contribute to the high prevalence of long-term cognitive, learning, and behavioral disability in survivors? *Pediatrics, 120*(3), 584.

Limperopoulos, C. J. (2008). Positive screening for autism in ex-preterm infants: Prevalence and risk factors. *Pediatrics, 121*(4), 758.

Lingam, R., Simmons, A., Andrews, N., Miller, E., Stowe, J., & Taylor, B. (2003). Prevalence of autism and parentally reported triggers in a north east London population. *Archives of Disease in Childhood, 88*(8), 666–670.

Liu, L. L., et al. (2010). Prevalence of overweight and obesity in youth with diabetes in USA: The SEARCH for Diabetes in Youth Study. *Pediatric Diabetes, 11*(1), 4–11. doi:10.1111/j.1399-5448.2009.00519.xx

Lyons, A. S., & Petrucelli, R. J. (1987). *Medicine: An illustrated history*. New York: Abradale Press.

Madea, B., Mußhoff, F., & Berghaus, G. (2006). *Verkehrsmedizin. Fahreignung, Fahrsicherheit, Unfallrekonstruktion*. Köln: Deutscher Ärzte-Verlag.

Madsen, K. M., et al. (2002). A population-based study of measles, mumps, and rubella vaccination and autism. *New England Journal of Medicine, 347*(19), 1477–1482.

Madsen, K. M., et al. (2003). Thimerosal and the occurrence of autism: Negative ecological evidence from Danish population-based data. *Pediatrics, 112*, 604–606. doi:10.1542/peds.112.3.204

Makela, A., Nuorti, J., & Peltola, H. (2002). Neurologic disorders after measles-mumps-rubella vaccination. *Pediatrics, 110*(5), 957–963.

Markel, H. (2011, February 28). Life, liberty and the pursuit of vaccines. *New York Times*. Retrieved from www.nytimes.com

Markowitz, L., Dunne, E., Saraiya, M., Hershel, L., Harrell, C., & Unger, E. (2007). Quadrivalent human papillomavirus vaccine. *Morbidity and Mortality Weekly, 56*(RR02), 1–24.

Marks, A., et al. (2010). Organophosphate pesticide exposure and attention in young Mexican-American children: The CHAMACOS Study. *Environmental Health Perspectives, 118*(12), 1768–1774.

Martin, B. J. (2008, October 30). TAP's patent application to give Lupron to autistic children. *Pathophilia*. [Weblog]. Retrieved from http:bmartinmd.com/2008/10/taps-patent-application-to-giv.html

Maryland State Board of Physicians. (2011, May 16). *Charges under the Maryland Medical Practices Act, case numbers 2008-0022 and 2009-0318*. Retrieved from www.mbp.state.md.us/BPQAPP/orders/GeierCharge05162011.pdf

Mayo Clinic. (2011, February 3). Precocious puberty: Treatment and drugs. Retrieved from www.mayoclinic.com/health/precocious-puberty/DS00883/DSECTION=treatments-and-drugs

Mayo Clinic. (2011, May 6). Obesity: Causes. Retrieved from www.mayoclinic.com/health/obesity/DS00314/DSECTION=causes

McCormack, M. C., et al. (2009). In-home particle concentrations and childhood asthma morbidity. *Environmental Health Perspectives, 117*(2), 294–298.

McKeever, T. M., Lewis, S. A., Smith, C., & Hubbard, R. (2004). Vaccination and allergic disease: A birth cohort study. *American Journal of Public Health,* 94(6), 985–989.

Merck & Co., Inc. (2009, January 09). Merck & Co., Inc. receives complete response letter from the Food and Drug Administration for use of Gardasil in women ages 27 through 45. Retrieved from www.businesswire.com

Mestel, R. (2002, December 15). Smallpox ravaged world for eons. *Los Angeles Times.* Retrieved from http:articles.latimes.com/2002/dec/15/science/sci-poxhistory15/2

Miller, J. (1998). *Becoming Laura Ingalls Wilder: The woman behind the legend.* Columbia: University of Missouri Press.

Mills, S., & Jones, T. (2009, May 21). Physician team's crusade shows cracks. *Chicago Tribune.* Retrieved from www.chicagotribune.com

Mitka, M. (2008). Chelation therapy trials halted. *Journal of the American Medical Association, 300*(19), 2236.

Mnookin, S. (2011). *The panic virus: A true story of medicine, science, and fear.* New York: Simon & Schuster.

Mokdad, A. H., et al. (2001). The continuing increase of diabetes in the U.S. *Diabetes Care, 24,* 412; doi:10.2337/diacare.24.2.412

Montague, B. (2006, February 22). Lady Mary Wortley Montagu, 1689–1762. The Montague Millennium. Retrieved from www.montaguemillennium.com/familyresearch/h_1762_mary.htm

Moore, K., et al. (2008). Ambient ozone concentrations cause increased hospitalizations for asthma in children: An 18-year study in southern California. *Environmental Health Perspectives, 116*(8), 1063–1070.

Muhle, R., Trentacoste, S. V., & Rapin, I. (2004). The genetics of autism. *Pediatrics, 113*(5), E472–E486.

Munoz, D. P., Armstrong, I. T., Hampton, K. A., & Moore, K. D. (2003). Altered control of visual fixation and saccadic eye movements in attention-deficit hyperactivity disorder. *Journal of Neurophysiology, 90,* 503–514.

Murch, S. H., et al. (2004). Retraction of an interpretation. *The Lancet, 363*(9411), 750.

Nadig, A. S., Ozonoff, S., Young, G. S., Rozga, A. Sigman, M., & Rogers, S. (2007). A prospective study of response to name in infants at risk for autism. *Archives of Pediatric and Adolescent Medicine, 161,* 378–383.

National Cancer Institute. (2011, September 9). Human papillomavirus (HPV) vaccines. Retrieved from www.cancer.gov/cancertopics/factsheet/prevention/HPV-vaccine

National Cancer Institute. (n.d.). NCI health information tip sheet for writers: Cancer health disparities. Retrieved from www.cancer.gov/newscenter/entertainment/tipsheet/cancer-health-disparities

National Cervical Cancer Coalition. (n.d.). What is the National Cervical Cancer Coalition? Retrieved from www.nccc-online.org/

National Institutes of Mental Health. (2007). Brain matures a few years late in ADHD, but follows normal pattern. Retrieved from www.nih.gov/news/pr/nov2007/nimh -12.htm

National Network for Immunization Information. (2008, March 3). Why is hepatitis B vaccination recommended for all infants, children, and adolescents? Retrieved from www.immunizationinfo.org/issues/general/why-hepatitis-b-immunization -recommended-all-infants-children-and-adolescents

National Network for Immunization Information. (2008, December 16). Pertussis (whooping cough): Understanding the disease. Retrieved from www.immunization info.org/vaccines/pertussis-whooping-cough

National Network for Immunization Information. (2009, July 16). Varicella: Understanding the disease. Retrieved from www.immunizationinfo.org/vaccines/ varicella-chickenpox

National Network for Immunization Information. (2010). Vaccine effectiveness: Do vaccines work? Retrieved from www.immunizationinfo.org/parents/why-immunize

National Network for Immunization Information. (n.d.). About NNii: Funding. Retrieved from www.immunizationinfo.org/about-nnii/funding

National Vaccine Information Center. (2009, February). An Analysis by the National Vaccine Information Center of Gardasil and Menactra adverse event reports to the Vaccine Adverse Events Reporting System (VAERS). Retrieved from www.nvic .org/Downloads/NVICGardasilvsMenactraVAERSReportFeb-2009u.aspx

National Vaccine Information Center. (n.d.). About National Vaccine Information Center. Retrieved from www.nvic.org/about.aspx#

Nelson, K., & Bauman, M. (2003). Thimerosal and autism. *Pediatrics, 111*(3). 674–679.

Neu, A., Kehrer, M., Hub, R., & Ranke, M. B. (1997). Incidence of type 1 diabetes in Germany is not higher than predicted: Response. *Diabetes Care, 20*(11), 1799–1800.

New York State Department of Health. (2010, October). Mumps. Retrieved from www.health.ny.gov/diseases/communicable/mumps/fact_sheet.htm

New York Times. (2008, September 9). Debunking an autism theory. *New York Times.* Retrieved from www.nytimes.com

Nilsson, L., Kjellman, N. I. M., & Bjorksten, B. (1998). A randomized controlled trial of the effect of pertussis vaccines on atopic disease. *Archives of Pediatric and Adolescent Medicine, 152*(8), 734–738.

Nilsson, L., Kjellman, N. I. M., & Bjorksten, B. (2003). Allergic disease at the age of 7 years after pertussis vaccination in infancy. *Archives of Pediatric and Adolescent Medicine, 157*(12), 1184–1189.

Offit, P. (2005). Why are pharmaceutical companies gradually abandoning vaccines? *Health Affairs, 24*(3), 622–630.

Offit, P. A. (2008). *Autism's false prophets: Bad science, risky medicine, and the search for a cure.* New York: Columbia University Press.

Offit, P. A. (2010). *Deadly choices: How the anti-vaccine movement threatens us all.* New York: Basic Books.

Offit, P., & Jew, R. (2003). Addressing parents' concerns: Do vaccines contain harmful preservatives, adjuvants, additives or residuals? *Pediatrics, 112*(6), 1394–1397.

Offit, P. A., & Hackett, C. J. (2003). Addressing parents' concerns: Do vaccines cause allergic or autoimmune diseases? *Pediatrics, 111*(3), 653–660. doi:10.1542/peds.111.3.653

Olmstead, D. (n.d.). A letter from the editor. *Age of Autism.* Retrieved from www.ageofautism.com/a-welcome-from-dan-olmste.html

Osterling, J., & Dawson, G. (1994). Early recognition of children with autism: A study of first birthday home videotapes. *Journal of Autism and Developmental Disorders, 24*(3), 247–257.

Paavonen, J., et al. (2009). Efficacy of human papillomavirus (HPV)-16/18 AS04-adjuvanted vaccine against cervical infection and precancer caused by oncogenic HPV types (PATRICIA): Final analysis of a double-blind, randomised study in young women. *The Lancet, 374*(9686), 301–314. doi:10.1016/S0140-6736(09)61248-4

Packard, J. M. (1999). *Victoria's daughters.* New York St. Martin's Griffin.

Park, R. L. (2001). *Voodoo science: The road from foolishness to fraud.* Oxford, UK: Oxford University Press.

Parker, S. K., Schwartz, B., Todd, J., & Pickering, L. K. (2004). Thimerosal-containing vaccines and autistic spectrum disorder: A critical review of published original data. *Pediatrics, 114,* 793–804.

Pascual, B., McGinley, E., Zanardi, L., Cortese, M., & Murphy, T. (2003). Tetanus surveillance 1998–2000. *Morbidity and Mortality Weekly, 52*(SS03), 1–8.

Peltola, H., Patja, A., Leinikki, P., Valle, M., Davidkin, I., & Paunio, M. (1998). No evidence for measles, mumps, and rubella vaccine-associated inflammatory bowel disease or autism in a 14-year prospective study. *The Lancet, 351*(9112), 1327.

Perlin, D., & Cohen, A. (2002). *The complete idiot's guide to dangerous diseases and epidemics.* New York: Alpha Books.

Pichichero, M. E., et al. (2008). Mercury levels in newborns and infants after receipt of thimerosal-containing vaccines. *Pediatrics, 121*(2), 208–214.

Pontifical Academy for Life. (2005, July 26). Vatican official clarifies stance on vaccines from fetal tissue. Retrieved from www.lifesitenews.com/news/archive/ldn/1950/72/5072604

Price, C. S., et al. (2010). Prenatal and infant exposure to thimerosal from vaccines and immunoglobulins and risk of autism. *Pediatrics, 126*(4), 656–664.

Prometheus. (2006, March 12). Armchair science vs. real science. [Weblog]. Retrieved from photoninthedarkness.blogspot.com/2006/03/armchair-science-vs-real-science.html

Racaniello, V. R. (2006). One hundred years of poliovirus pathogenesis. *Virology, 344*(1), 9–16. doi:10.1016/j.virol.2005.09.015

Rathore, M., & Mirza, A. (2010, July 8). Pediatric haemophilus influenzae infection. Retrieved from http:emedicine.medscape.com/article/964317-overview#showall

Reibel, K. (2008, January 30). Autism and the Amish. Retrieved from http:autism-news-beat.com/archives/29

Reinberg, S. (2011, August 9). CDC urges all Americans to get flu shots. *USA Today.* Retrieved from http:yourlife.usatoday.com/

Reproductive Health Outlook: Cervical Cancer. (n.d.). About cervical cancer. Retrieved from www.rho.org/about-cervical-cancer.htm

Research Autism. (2011, July 11). Chelation and autism. Retrieved from www.researchautism.net/autism_treatments_therapies_intervention.ikml?ra=25

Riedel, S. (2005). Edward Jenner and the history of smallpox and vaccination. *Baylor University Medical Center Proceedings, 18*(1), 21–25.

Rocky Mountain News. (2008, March 10). No link to autism: Settlement fails to strengthen case against vaccinations. *Rocky Mountain News.*

Roost, H. P., et al. (2004). Influence of MMR-vaccinations and diseases on atopic sensitization and allergic symptoms in Swiss schoolchildren. *Pediatric Allergy and Immunology, 15*(5), 401–407. doi:10.1111/j.1399-3038.2004.00192.x

Roush, S. W., & Murphy, T. V. (2007). Historical comparisons of morbidity and mortality for vaccine-preventable diseases in the United States. *Journal of the American Medical Association, 298*(18), 2155–2163.

Royland, F. D. (2011, May 20). O'Malley ousts David Geier from autism commission. *Baltimore Sun.* Retrieved from www.baltimoresun.com

Rubia, K., Smith, A. B., Brammer, M. J., Toone, B., & Taylor, E. (2005). Abnormal brain activation during inhibition and error detection in medication-naïve adolescents with ADHD. *American Journal of Psychiatry, 162*(6), 1067–1075.

Schechter, R., & Grether, J. K. (2008). Continuing increases in autism reported to California developmental services system: Mercury in retrograde. *Archives of General Psychiatry, 65*(1), 19–24.

Schiffman, M., & Castle, P. E. (2003). Human papillomavirus: Epidemiology and public health. *Archives of Pathology and Laboratory Medicine, 127*(8), 930–934.

Schiffman, M., Castle, P. E., Jeronimo, J., Rodriguez, A. C., & Wacholder, S. (2007). Human papillomavirus and cervical cancer. *The Lancet, 370,* 9590.

Schlenker, B., et al. (2011). Intermediate-differentiated invasive (pT1 G2) penile cancer—oncological outcome and follow-up. *Urologic Oncology, 29*(6), 782–787. doi:10.1016/j.urolonc.2009.08.022

Schumann, C. M., et al. (2004). The amygdala is enlarged in children but not adolescents with autism; the hippocampus is enlarged at all ages. *Journal of Neuroscience, 24*(28), 6392–6401. doi:10.1523/JNEUROSCI.1297-04.2004

Serene, J., Ashtari, M., Szeszko, P. R., & Kumra, S. (2007). Neuroimaging studies of children with serious emotional disturbances: A selective review. *Canadian Journal of Psychiatry, 52*(3), 135–145.

Shattuck, P. T. (2006). The contribution of diagnostic substitution to the growing administrative prevalence of autism in U.S. special education. *Pediatrics, 117*(4), 1028–1037. doi:10.1542/peds.2005-1516

Shaw, P., et al. (2007). Attention-deficit/hyperactivity disorder is characterized by a delay in cortical maturation. *Proceedings of the National Academy of Sciences of the United States of America, 104*(49), 19649–19654.

Shelton, J. F., Tancredi, D. J., & Hertz-Picciotto, I. (2010). Independent and dependent contributions of advanced maternal and paternal ages to autism risk. *Autism Research, 3,* 30–39.

Shermer, M. (2002). *Why people believe weird things: Pseudoscience, superstition, and other confusions of our time.* New York: Holt.

Siedel, K. (2006, June 20). An elusive institute [Weblog]. Retrieved from http:neurodiversity.com/weblog/article/98/an-elusive-institute-significant-misrepre sentations-mark-geier-david-geier-the-evolution-of-the-lupron-protocol-part-two

Siegel, B., Pliner, C., Eschler, J., & Elliot, G. R. (1988). How children with autism are diagnosed: Difficulties in identification of children with multiple developmental delays. *Developmental and Behavioral Pediatrics, 9*(4), 199–204.

Silverman, C., & Brosco, J. P. (2007). Understanding autism: Parents and pediatricians in historical perspective. *Archives of Pediatric and Adolescent Medicine, 161,* 392–398.

Smeeth, L., et al. (2004). MMR vaccination and pervasive developmental disorders: A case-control study. *The Lancet, 364*(9438), 963–969.

Smith, B. (2012, February). Dr. Merola: Visionary or quack? *Chicago Magazine.*

Smith, J. S. (1991). *Patenting the sun: Polio and the Salk vaccine.* New York: Anchor Books.

Smith, M., & Woods, C. (2010). On-time vaccine receipt in the first year does not adversely affect neuropsychological outcomes. *Pediatrics, 125*(6), 1134–1141.

Smith, M. E., & Gevins, A. (2004). Attention and brain activity while watching television: Components of viewer engagement. *Media Psychology, 6,* 285–305.

Soltesz, G. G., Patterson, C. C., & Dahlquist, G. G. (2007). Worldwide childhood type 1 diabetes incidence—what can we learn from epidemiology? *Pediatric Diabetes, 8,* 6–14. doi:10.1111/j.1399-5448.2007.00280.x

Sowell, E. R., Thompson, P. M., Welcome, S. E., Henkenius, A. L., Toga, A. W., & Peterson, B. S. (2003). Cortical abnormalities in children and adolescents with attention-deficit hyperactivity disorder. *The Lancet, 362*(9397), 1699–1707.

State, M. W. (2010). The genetics of child psychiatric disorders: Focus on autism and Tourette syndrome. *Neuron, 68*(2), 254–269. doi:10.1016/j.neuron.2010.10.004

Steckelberg, J. (2010, December 16). What happens if you get tetanus shots too close together—within a few years instead of the recommended 10 years? Retrieved from www.mayoclinic.com/health/tetanus-shots/AN01497

Stevens, T., & Mulsow, M. (2006). There is no meaningful relationship between television exposure and symptoms of attention-deficit/hyperactivity disorder. *Pediatrics, 117,* 665–672. doi:10.1542/peds.2005-0863

Stobbe, M. (2010, February 7). Millions of swine flu vaccine doses to be burned. *USA Today.* Retrieved from www.usatoday.com

Stoppard, M. (2009, October 12). Why we're too ready to call people autistic. *Mirror.* Retrieved from www.thefreelibrary.com

Stöppler, M. C. (2009, April 16). Cervical dysplasia. Retrieved from www.medicinenet .com/cervical_dysplasia/article.htm

Strachan, D. P. (1989). Hayfever, hygiene, and household size. *British Journal of Medicine, 299,* 1259–1269.

Stratton, K., Gable, A., & McCormick, M. C. (Eds.). (2001). Immunization safety review: Thimerosal-containing vaccines and neurodevelopmental disorders. Washington, DC: National Academy Press.

Sugerman, D. E., et al. (2010). Measles outbreak in a highly vaccinated population, San Diego 2008: Role of the unintentionally unvaccinated. *Pediatrics, 125*(4), 747–755.

Szatmari, P., et al. (2007). Mapping autism risk loci using genetic linkage and chromosomal rearrangements. *Nature Genetics, 39*(3), 319–328.

Taylor, B., et al. (1999). Autism and measles, mumps, and rubella vaccine: No epidemiological evidence for a causal association. *The Lancet, 353*(9169), 2026–2029.

Terbush, J. (2011, September 13). Does the HPV vaccine really cause retardation? *Business Insider.* Retrieved from www.businessinsider.com

Texas House of Representatives. HB 1098. Retrieved from www.legis.state.tx.us/tlodocs/80R/billtext/html/HB01098F.htm

Thigpen, M. C., et al. (2011). Bacterial meningitis in the United States 1998–2007. *New England Journal of Medicine, 364*(21), 2016–2025.

Thompson, W. W., et al. (2007). Early thimerosal exposure and neuropsychological outcomes at 7 to 10 years. *New England Journal of Medicine, 357*(13), 1281–1292.

Todar, K. (n.d.). Diphtheria. *Todar's online textbook of biology.* Retrieved from www.textbookofbacteriology.net/diphtheria.html

Tran, T. (2009). Management of hepatitis B in pregnancy: Weighing the options. *Cleveland Clinic Journal of Medicine, 76,* 525–529.

U.S. Department of Health and Human Services. (2008, September). Aluminum CAS # 7429-90-5. Agency for Toxic Substances and Disease Registry. Division of Toxicology and Environmental Medicine. Retrieved from www.atsdr.cdc.gov/tfacts22.pdf

U.S. Department of Health and Human Services. (n.d.). About the VAERS program. Retrieved from http:vaers.hhs.gov/about/index

U.S. Department of Health and Human Services. (n.d.). VAERS data. Retrieved from http:vaers.hhs.gov/data/index

U.S. Food and Drug Administration. (2009, March 3). Institutional review boards frequently asked questions—information sheet. Retrieved from www.fda.gov/RegulatoryInformation/Guidances/ucm126420.htm

U.S. National Library of Medicine. (2011, December 9). Smallpox: A great and terrible scourge. Retrieved from www.nlm.nih.gov/exhibition/smallpox/sp_threat.html

Uchiyama, T., Kurosawa, M., & Inaba, Y. (2007). MMR-vaccine and regression in autism spectrum disorders: Negative results presented from Japan. *Journal of Autism and Developmental Disorders, 37*(2), 210–217.

USA Today. (2010, February 16). Vaccine fear-mongering endangers child health. *USA Today.* Retrieved from www.usatoday.com

Vaccine Education Center at the Children's Hospital of Philadelphia. (2009, Spring). Aluminum in vaccines: What you should know. Retrieved from www.chop.edu/export/download/pdfs/articles/vaccine-education-center/aluminum.pdf

Vaccine Education Center at the Children's Hospital of Philadelphia. (2011, October). Hot topics: Aluminum. Retrieved from www.chop.edu/service/vaccine-education-center/hot-topics/aluminum.html

Vasilakopoulou, A. A., & le Roux, C. W. (2007). Could a virus contribute to weight gain? *International Journal of Obesity, 31*(9), 1350–1356. doi:10.1038/sj.ijo.0803623

Verreault, R., Laurin, D., Lindsay, J., & De Serres, G. (2001). Past exposure to vaccines and subsequent risk of Alzheimer's disease. *Canadian Medical Association Journal, 165*(11), 1495–1498.

Wakefield, A. J., & Fundenberg, H. (1998, April 6). U.K. patent application GB 2 325 856 A. Retrieved from http:briandeer.com/mmr/1998-vaccine-patent.pdf

Wakefield, A. J., et al. (1998). Ileal-lymphoid-nodular hyperplasia, non-specific colitis, and pervasive developmental disorder in children. *The Lancet, 351,* 637–641.

Walboomers, J. M. M., et al. (1999). Human papillomavirus is a necessary cause of invasive cervical cancer worldwide. *Journal of Pathology, 189*(1), 12–19.

Wallis, C. (2009, November 3). A powerful identity, a vanishing diagnosis. *New York Times.* Retrieved from www.nytimes.com

WebMD. (2004, December 8). RxList: Neomycin sulfate indications and dosage. Retrieved from www.rxlist.com/neomycin_sulfate-drug.htm

WebMD. (2009, June 30). Chelation therapy: Topic overview. Retrieved from www.webmd.com/balance/tc/chelation-therapy-topic-overview

Whitmore, C. (2010). Type 2 diabetes and obesity in adults. *British Journal of Nursing, 19*(14), 880–886.

Willingham, E. J. (2011, May 5). Autism, Lupron, the Geiers, and what can science do about emotions? *Science, Society, and You.* [Weblog]. Retrieved from http:biology files.fieldofscience.com/2011/05/autism-lupron-geiers-and-what-can.html

World Health Organization. (2006). WHO position paper on haemophilus influenzae type b conjugate vaccines. *Weekly Epidemiology Record, 81*(47), 445–452.

World Health Organization. (2006, July 10). About WHO. Retrieved from https://apps.who.int/aboutwho/en/achievements.html

World Health Organization. (2008, August). Hepatitis B fact sheet. Retrieved from www.who.int/mediacentre/factsheets/fs204/en/

World Health Organization. (2011, May 21). Smallpox. Retrieved from www.who.int/mediacentre/factsheets/smallpox/en/

World Health Organization. (2011, July 14). WPRO scarlet fever update. Retrieved from www.wpro.who.int/health_topics/scarlet_fever/

World Health Organization. (2011, August 4). Obesity and overweight fact sheet. Retrieved from www.who.int/mediacentre/factsheets/fs311/en/

World Health Organization. (2011, September 23). Diphtheria reported cases. Retrieved from http:apps.who.int/immunization_monitoring/en/globalsummary/time series/tsincidencedip.htm

Yeargin-Allsopp, M., Rice, C., Karapurkar, R., Doernberg, N., Boyle, C., & Murphy. C. (2003). Prevalence of autism in a US metropolitan area. *Journal of the American Medical Association, 289*(1), 49–55.

Yirmiya, N., & Charman, T. (2010). The prodrome of autism: Early behavioral and biological signs, regression, peri- and post-natal development and genetics. *Journal of Child Psychology and Psychiatry, 51*(4), 432–458. doi:10.1111/j.1469-7610.2010.02214

Index

About the Authors

Stacy Mintzer Herlihy is a freelance writer. Her articles have appeared in many publications such as *USA Today* and *Today's Parent*. In between writing assignments, Ms. Herlihy grades nationally standardized tests at home online. She lives in New Jersey with her husband, two kids, and fifteen-pound Maine Coon cat, Lucy. This is her first book.

E. Allison Hagood is a community college psychology professor. Before becoming a professor, she was a clinician and researcher specializing in adults with severe mental illnesses. She is a member of the American Psychological Association, the Association for Psychological Science, and the Society for the Teaching of Psychology.

CPSIA information can be obtained at www.ICGtesting.com
Printed in the USA
BVOW04s1628110115

382709BV00002B/3/P